CONDITIONING FOR BASEBALL
Pre-season
Regular Season
and
Off-season

CONDITIONING FOR BASEBALL

Pre-season

Regular Season

and

Off-season

By

ROBERT R. SPACKMAN JR., M.S., R.P.T.

Athletic Trainer
Assistant Professor of Physical Education
Southern Illinois University
Carbondale, Illinois

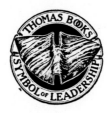

CHARLES C THOMAS • **PUBLISHER**
Springfield · Illinois · U.S.A.

Published and Distributed Throughout the World by

CHARLES C THOMAS • PUBLISHER

Bannerstone House

301-327 East Lawrence Avenue, Springfield, Illinois, U.S.A.

Natchez Plantation House

735 North Atlantic Boulevard, Fort Lauderdale, Florida, U.S.A.

With **THOMAS BOOKS** *careful attention is given to all details of
manufacturing and design. It is the Publisher's desire to present books
that are satisfactory as to their physical qualities and artistic possibilities
and appropriate for their particular use.* **THOMAS BOOKS** *will be true
to those laws of quality that assure a good name and good will.*

Printed in the United States of America

E-1

Dedicated to my wife, Jane,
and to my four children

Acknowledgments

The author wishes to express his sincere appreciation to those who gave freely of their time and assistance in helping with this book. Special thanks are due to Mrs. Claudeis Selby, English Department, Southern Illinois University, for her assistance and help in preparing the manuscript.

The author is indebted to Fred Orlofsky, Charles Ehrlich, Craig Anderson and Bill Lepsi who kindly consented to pose and demonstrate the exercises for the pictures in the book. Fred Orlofsky and Charles Ehrlich were outstanding gymnasts at Southern Illinois University. Craig Anderson is a pitcher for the New York "Mets" baseball team, and Bill Lepsi is a football player for the Kansas City "Chiefs" football team.

The author wishes to express appreciation to Robert "Rip" Stokes for his suggestions and help in the photography used in the manuscript.

R.R.S.

Contents

CONDITIONING FOR BASEBALL

Pre-season
Regular Season
and
Off-season

Introduction

This conditioning program for the baseball player has been designed as a complete program for the whole year. The exercises are divided into pre-season, season and off-season programs. To condition the body completely, a program must include warm-up exercises, stretching exercises for flexibility, resistive exercises for strength and cardiovascular exercises for endurance.

Many baseball players do not know how to condition their bodies. This program can be used by all individual participants, managers, physical education instructors and coaches from the little leagues to major leagues. Trainers, managers and coaches can mark the exercises they want their players to be sure to do in order to strengthen a weak arm, back or leg.

Each baseball player, however, should do the stretching exercises, strengthening exercises, cardiovascular exercises and the isometric exercises. Each player should then continue his conditioning by following the sprinting exercises suggested for his individual position. Each player naturally will condition a little differently, depending upon the demands of the position he will be playing.

With isometric exercise expensive equipment is not needed. Two players can work together and strengthen the whole body. Start with only a few exercises the first day. Gradually increase the number of repetitions and the number of exercises as your physical condition improves.

Baseball is a game which requires many short sprints and short bursts of energy. As a result, there are many injuries due to poor general physical condition, cooling off during the game and just letting yourself get out of condition during the season.

Follow the exercise directions closely to be sure you do them correctly. Exercises done incorrectly or spasmotically will not produce the desired results. It is important to follow the seasonal program in order to stay in good physical condition during the long season.

During the off-season, try to work out for an hour to an hour and a half at least three days a week. Every other day is best. Follow the recommended program and play some other sport to keep your weight down and maintain your cardiovascular condition. Handball and swimming are two of the best all-around conditioners. Many baseball players play golf. This is fine provided you also do something else more strenuous.

At least thirty days before spring training or practice begins, begin your pre-season conditioning and work out seven days a week. Some of the heavier players may need six to eight weeks of pre-season conditioning to get their weight down to desirable playing weight.

CONDITIONING FOR BASEBALL

A majority of today's baseball players are not really well-conditioned athletes. Many of them are a little lazy, and since the game itself consists of short sprints, there is time to catch your breath between efforts. Some baseball men think that specific exercises are not necessary and that they can play themselves into condition during spring practice. We know they cannot play themselves into good physical condition because of the limited physical demands of the game itself. Many players also have old injuries and weak areas in the body which require specific attention. No doubt there would be fewer baseball injuries in the first place if players were truly well conditioned.

The only players on most professional teams, or on any organized teams, who are in top physical condition are the pitchers, and the coaches usually "run" them into condition. The only other players who may stay in condition by playing are the .300 hitters who get on base every day. The rest of the players seldom are in good physical condition; consequently there is a high percentage of injuries and too many players with talent that never have that good year or reach their potential.

How many times during a year do you see a player hit a triple and be winded for five minutes, not being able to catch his breath? The next hitter may hit a fly ball, and our runner is too winded to score from third base. In double headers, many players do not hustle on that ground ball back to the pitcher or take the extra base during the second game because of fatigue. How often we see the player who is zero for four times at bat after two strike outs and two pop flies! He has not run hard all day, and then he hits a double down the foul line. He rounds first base and pulls a muscle going into second base because he did not sprint hard on the pop flies and because he did not keep his legs warm by sprinting in and out from his position when the teams changed positions.

Only the great athletes hustle every day on every play. Indeed, most athletes are a little lazy and will only do as much as the coach or manager requires them to do. To make matters worse, many athletes and coaches do not know how to get in top physical condition or how to remain in good physical condition all season.

Conditioning is a year-round necessity if you want to be a good athlete. There is no reason for baseball players to end a career at thirty or even forty years of age if their bodies are conditioned twelve months a year.

EXERCISE AND THE ATHLETE

It is now generally accepted that the competitor must stay in good condition all year long; he cannot be a seasonal athlete. There was a time, not too many years ago, when most athletes competed in two, three and even more sports each year. We now live in an age of specialization, and only a few boys compete in more than two sports. This means the athlete must somehow stay in good physical condition for twelve months a year. An isometric program can maintain the strength of every baseball player in the off-season. Always

work out at least three days a week in the off-season to maintain your physical condition.

Many professional, college and high school baseball players condition for the sport season only and then allow themselves to get sadly out of condition in the off-season. Each year as he ages the athlete gets further out of condition in the off-season and has a more difficult time reconditioning at the beginning of a new season.

STRETCHING EXERCISES

Every good athlete must have strength, endurance, speed, agility, cardiovascular endurance and flexibility. Flexibility in the back, chest, shoulders, arms and legs is an absolute necessity for baseball players. All baseball players who throw and run well are flexible.

Here are a few simple tests to see whether you are loose or tight. With the knees straight, you should be able to lay your palms flat on the floor. Lying on your back, you should be able to be comfortable with no tightness in the chest, with your arms overhead and flat on the floor. Baseball players should be able to lay their palms on the floor with their knees straight. If you cannot do this, you have tight hamstring muscles (back of the legs), tight low back muscles or both. Stretch daily until you can lay your palms flat on the floor.

Players who can throw well have great range of motion in external rotation of the shoulder. Should you be tight in any area, it is best to do your stretching in the shower room daily. See stretching exercises using shower-room procedure on page xx. Follow the stretching exercises daily using a fungo bat, or substitute a broom stick 42 in. to 46 in. long. Check your flexibility with the pictures on page 5.

STRENGTH TESTING

The baseball coach should be interested in a method of strength testing. With a two-man exercise program the coach or trainer can test the muscle strength of individual muscle groups. Each baseball squad requires different exercises. Design your program to the needs of your base-

Good range in external rotation.   Good range in internal rotation.

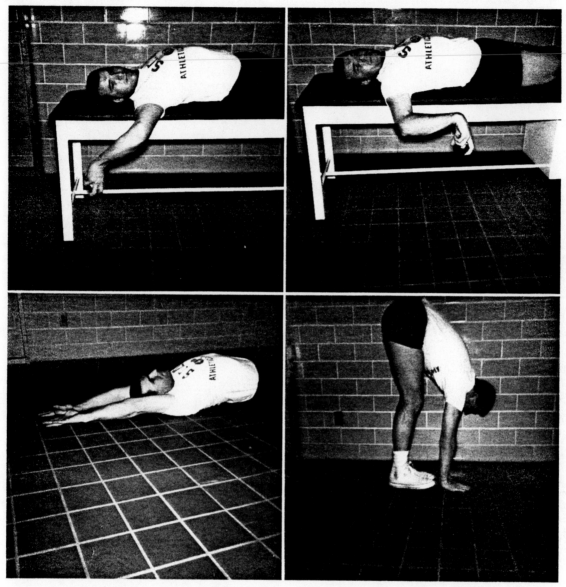

Arms flat on the floor overhead.   Can you lay your palms flat on the floor
                                     with your knees straight?

ball team. In general, all baseball players should have strong hands, arms, shoulders, back and legs, so include strength work in your daily practice in these areas.

In the off-season, mark the exercises in the book you want each individual baseball player to be sure to do to strengthen his weak knee, shoulder or other weak area. Each player will spend more time strengthening his own weak area. The whole squad will do all the exercises suggested for baseball players.

The baseball coach or trainer should give a strength test to his team every year to be sure last year's injured shoulder or leg is strong before beginning a new season. Know your team and try to prevent injuries rather than try to rehabilitate them after they occur.

By comparing the muscle strength of one

extremity with that on the other side, one can detect weakness to some degree. For example, to test the strength of the big muscles over the point of the shoulder (deltoids), see exercises 1, 2 and 3 under Shoulder and Arm Exercises on page 53. Where there is unequal strength when lifting the arms forward, the man giving the resistance can easily distinguish which arm is the weaker. Raise the arms to the side and resist; push the arms backward and resist. In this manner one can test the muscle strength of the deltoid group. Should there be a weakness, continue the exercise on both extremities until the strength appears to be the same. Then continue the exercise daily throughout the season to increase or maintain the strength.

No one knows what normal strength is in any area of the body or for any particular body weight. Due to variables such as age, weight, height, body build, length of the lever, previous activity or sports, diet and many others, we cannot set up norms.

Many baseball players have weak backs on one side because of previous injuries and the game itself with repeated sliding into bases and twisting of the back while hitting. To check strength in the lower back, see Back Exercises, numbers 6 and 7 on pages 65 and 66. It will be easy to determine muscle weakness to some degree. Continue the exercises until both sides of the back seem to have the same strength and there is no pain. Then continue the exercise daily throughout the season to increase or maintain the strength. You can test the muscle strength in the whole body by comparing the strength of one extremity with the other or one side of the body with the other side.

Muscle strength both before and after an exercise program can be best evaluated with strength testing equipment. There are many variables in manual strength testing, but where there is no testing apparatus, the comparison method described above appears to be the best. I now have a muscle testing device on the market—the Spackman Muscle Testing Unit. It is manufactured by La Berne Manufacturing Company (819 Leesburg Road, Columbia, S. C. 29205).

By testing muscle strength it is possible with my testing device to tell if the athlete is strong or weak. Should an injury occur, one can tell how much strength has been lost due to the injury.

Following a corrective exercise program a comparison can then be made of the results of the tests done before the injury. This way one can tell when he is back to normal strength. This device acts as a motivator to anyone who is interested in gaining muscle strength.

Off-season Conditioning

Wrist Roller

To strengthen the forearm and wrist, all baseball players should make this simple device and use it daily. Take an old baseball bat with a handle you like; an old broomstick will do. Cut the barrel (big end of the bat) off to a piece about 14 in. long. Drill a hole in the center of the bat handle. Cut a piece of rope 5 ft. long and thread is through the hole. Tie a brick or a weight on the end of the rope. See page 29.

Grasp the bat in the hands and hold it out at shoulder height. Slowly twist the bat and wind the rope in order to roll the brick up to the bat handle. Alternate one hand and then the other, reaching way under, and roll the wrist over the top very slowly. Slowly lower the weight the same way. Roll the weight up and down slowly five times daily. When five repetitions become an easy task, add another brick or more weight.

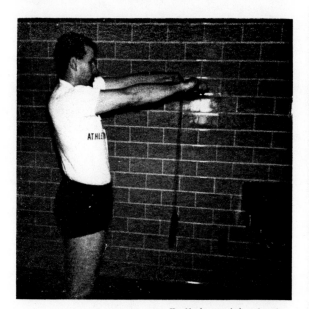 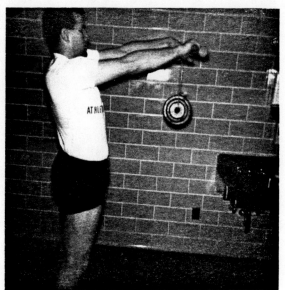

Roll the weight slowly up and down the bat handle.

Weighted Bat

Every baseball player should have a bat, his favorite model if possible, loaded with weight. This may be done yourself by drilling a 6-to 8-in. hole in the end of the bat and driving a piece of metal into the hole. You may also use melted lead to fill the hole in the bat. If you have no weighted bat, you may tie a brick or a weight on a broomstick or use a weighted bar.

The following wrist and forearm exercises should be done daily with the weighted bat in order to increase and maintain your strength. If the bat is too heavy, slide the hand up the handle and exercise from this position. As strength increases move the hand to the end of the bat. Exercise both arms and wrists. You should experience no pain during the exercise; if you

7

do, you have a weak or injured wrist. Should you have pain during exercises, you will keep the wrist sore, and it will remain weak. Slide your hand up the bat so that you can exercise without pain. See exercises on page 28.

Swinging a weighted bat can be dangerous unless you are thoroughly warmed up, loose and have no muscle tightness in the shoulders. It is true that many players swing a weighted bat in the hitter's circle before they hit, but they are usually loose and the weather is warm or even hot during the baseball season. It is better to use the weighted bat to strengthen and stretch the muscles, but swing only your favorite model of the weight you like. Exercise with the weighted bat both in the off-season and daily during the regular season in order to maintain your strength.

Medi Exercise Ball

Medi exercise ball.

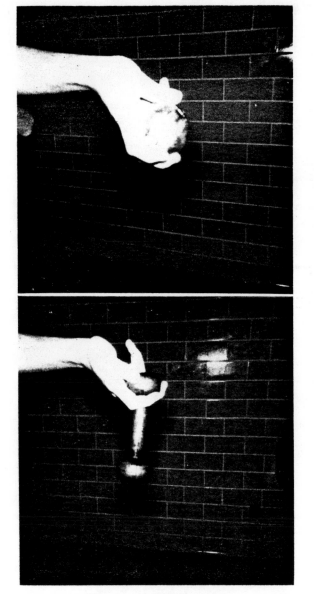

Four-pound solid dumbbell.

If you want to be good at anything, you have to work at it constantly. Every baseball player should have a metal baseball to strengthen and stretch the muscles of the shoulder, forearm, wrist, chest and back.

You can purchase a medi exercise ball from Van Sickle Company, 2115 59th Street, St. Louis 10, Missouri, for $6.00. The medi exercise ball is a moulded baseball that weighs between 3 and 4 lbs. If you are handy, perhaps you can make your own metal baseball or use a 3- of 4-lb. solid dumbbell.

These exercises were originated by Bob Bauman, trainer with the St. Louis "Cardinals" baseball team. Bob has rehabilitated and strengthened more baseball players' arms than any trainer in the country. The author had the pleasure of working for Bob Bauman for several years when he was head trainer for the old St. Louis "Browns" in the American League.

The following exercises should be done with both arms in the off-season and daily with the throwing arm during the regular season.

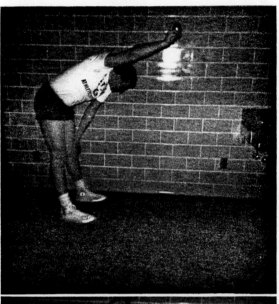

Forward swing.

1. Forward and Backward Swings

a. Place the left hand on the left knee and bend forward at the waist. The feet are spread apart about 24 in.

b. Grasp the ball in the right hand with the arm hanging loosely in front of the body.

c. Swing the ball forward overhead and backward, letting the ball carry the arm.

d. Repeat ten to twenty forward and backward swings.

e. Repeat the same exercise raising the ball forward and backward very slowly five times, getting a good stretch in each direction.

f. Repeat the exercise with the left arm.

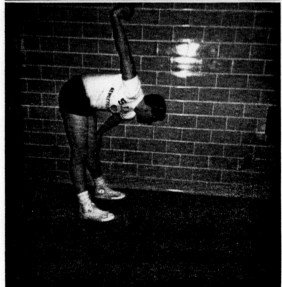

Backward swing.

Lateral swing across the chest.

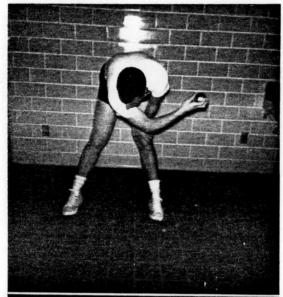

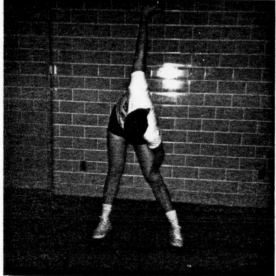

Lateral swing back to the right.

2. Lateral Swing Side to Side

   a. Place the left hand on the left knee and bend forward at the waist. The feet are spread apart about 24 in.

   b. Grasp the ball in the right hand with the arm hanging loosely in front of the body.

   c. Swing the ball across the chest to the left and back up to the right, letting the ball carry the arm.

   d. Repeat ten to twenty lateral swings from side to side.

   e. Repeat the same exercise raising the ball from side to side very slowly five times, getting a good stretch in each direction.

   f. Repeat the exercise with the left arm.

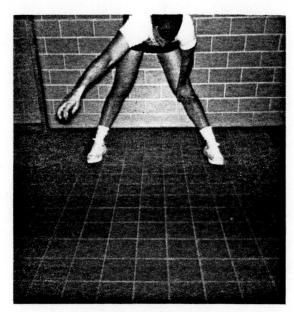

Circle swing to the right.

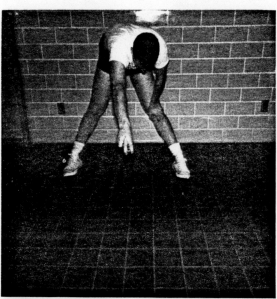

Circle swing forward.

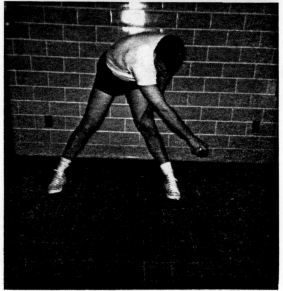

Circle swing to the left.

3. Circle Swing

a. Place the left hand on the left knee and bend forward at the waist. The feet are spread apart about 24 in.

b. Grasp the ball in the right hand with the arm hanging loosely in front of the body.

c. Swing the ball, making a circle in a clockwise direction for ten circles. Swing the ball in a circle counterclockwise direction for ten circles.

d. Repeat the same exercise, making a clockwise circle very slowly five times. Repeat a counterclockwise circle very slowly five times, getting a good stretch in each direction.

e. Repeat the exercise with the left arm.

Starting position.

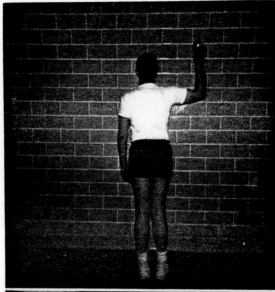

4. Overhead Stretch

a. Stand straight with the shoulders level, feet spread about 24 in. apart. Bend the elbow to 90 degrees and raise the arm to shoulder level.

b. Grasp the ball in the right hand in a perpendicular position.

c. Raise the ball straight upward, extending the elbow. Keep the shoulders level and push as high as possible, getting a good stretch along the arm and side of the chest.

d. Return to the starting position.

e. Repeat five to ten overhead stretches, trying to go a little higher on each stretch.

f. Repeat the exercise with the left arm.

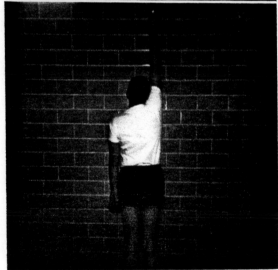

Overhead stretch.

Shoulder external rotation.

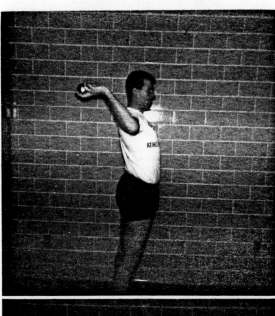

5. Shoulder Rotation (External and Internal)

a. Stand straight with the shoulders level, feet spread apart about 24 in. Bend the elbow to 90 degrees and raise the arm to shoulder level.

b. Grasp the ball in the right hand. Slowly rotate the arm externally as you do in throwing, bending the wrist backward. Get a good stretch in the shoulder.

c. Slowly rotate the arm internally as you do in throwing, bending the wrist forward. Keep the wrist and elbow at shoulder level. Get a good stretch in the shoulder.

d. Repeat external and internal rotation of the shoulder five times, getting a good stretch.

e. Repeat the exercise with the left arm.

f. Repeat the same exercise lying on a table, keeping the wrist and elbow at shoulder level while rotating the arm externally and internally stretching the shoulder.

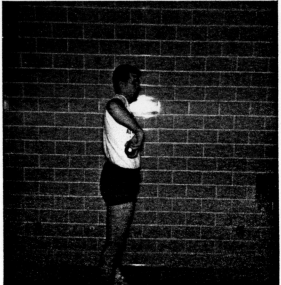

Shoulder internal rotation.

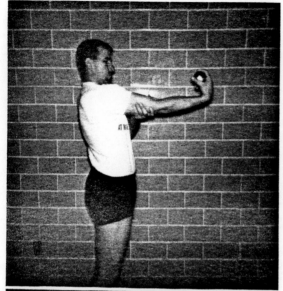

6. Biceps and Wrist Stretching and Strengthening

a. Stand straight with the shoulders level, feet spread about 24 in. apart. Raise the right arm to shoulder level with the palm up. The left hand is placed under the right upper arm to hold the shoulder and elbow level.

b. Grasp the ball in the right hand and slowly bend the wrist upward and downward, getting a good stretch. Slowly bend

Wrist flexion.

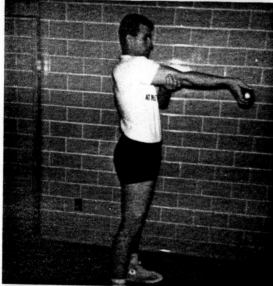

Wrist extension.

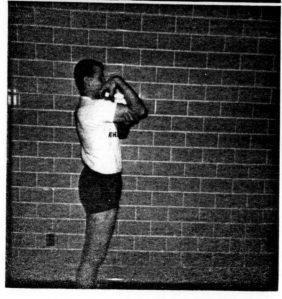

Elbow flexion.

the elbow upward and downward, getting a good stretch. Slowly rotate the forearm inwardly and outwardly (supination and pronation), getting a good stretch.

c. Repeat each exercise of the wrist, forearm and elbow five times, getting a good stretch.

d. Repeat the same exercise slowly with the left arm.

e. See the pictures on pages 14 and 15.

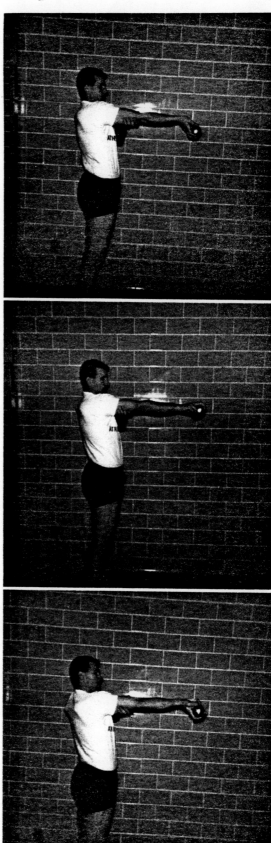

Elbow extension.

Wrist pronation (palm down).

Wrist supination (palm up).

CARDIOVASCULAR EXERCISE

Since baseball is a game of many short sprints and repeated short bursts of energy, every baseball player needs cardiovascular endurance. Here are four ways you can improve and maintain your cardiovascular endurance in the off-season and pre-season conditioning programs. These methods do not replace running; they just supplement running when you cannot get outside to run.

Make yourself a box or a stool 20 in high, 20 in. wide and 20 in. deep. This exercise is called "The Brouha Step Test"[1] or "The Harvard Step Test." In this exercise the player steps up and down on a 20 in. box thirty times a minute for five minutes. On the count of one, step up on the box with the left foot; step up with the right foot on the count of two; then step down with the left foot; and on the count of four, step down with the right foot. After two and one half minutes, change and lead with the right foot. As this exercise becomes easy, you may add weight to the feet, wear a weighted belt or hold dumbbells in each hand.

Pulse rates may be taken before and after exercise; improvement is shown by a lowered resting pulse rate after five minutes of exercise and by a quickened recovery to a resting pulse rate after five minutes of exercise.

In the first few days, when beginning the step test, you may start out at a cadence of twenty-four steps per minute for three minutes. When five minutes is easy at twenty-four steps per minute, step up the cadence to thirty steps per minute. See the pictures on page 17.

Another cardiovascular exercise you may do for developing endurance is known as "The Carlson Fatigue Test."[2] It is easier on the feet to do this exercise on a mat or on a soft surface.

The exercise consists of running in place as fast as you can for ten seconds, rest ten seconds; this is repeated for ten bouts—or the equivalent of ten 100-yd. dashes in ten seconds, with ten seconds rest between each dash. Count each time your right foot contacts the floor and record this number after each ten-second run. As a check on your progress, five measures of pulse rate are taken: (a) before exercises; (b) ten seconds after exercises; (c) two minutes after exercises; (d) four minutes after exercises; (e) six minutes after exercise. A quick return to normal pulse rate after exercise and an increase in number of times the right foot hits the floor give indications of your improvement in conditioning.

Rope skipping is another good cardiovascular exercise that may be done outdoors, or indoors in bad weather. There are many methods of skipping rope—alternating on one foot and then the other foot, on both feet or the boxer's shuffle as boxers skip rope. In this method you only jump high enough for the rope to clear your feet.

Timing your rope skipping is one method of measuring your improvement. Skip rope for one minute and rest for one minute. This may be repeated for ten one-minute periods with one-minute rest between. Should this become too easy, increase the number to fifteen one-minute periods or add weighted spats when skipping.

Pick ups. This is an old baseball stretching and cardiovascular drill that all players do in their pre-season conditioning. Pitchers always do much more of this drill than the other players. It may be done outdoors or indoors in the gym.

One player assumes an infielder's position, while a partner, standing 5 to 10 yds. away, rolls the ball. First the partner rolls the ball to your right so that you have to sprint and stretch to get to the ball. You field the ball and throw it back to your partner. Your partner then rolls the ball to your left, just hard enough so that you have to stretch again to get to the ball. The ball is thrown or rolled to the right and then to the left alternating until you are winded and scarcely can run for the next ball. You then change places, and your partner does the fielding while you roll the ball. As your cardiovascular condition improves, you can run and field the ball for a longer period, increasing your endurance.

This is an excellent drill incorporating running, stretching, twisting, bending and fielding. All players should do this drill pre-seasonally to increase their endurance.

[1] BROUHA, L.: The step test: A simple method of measuring physical fitness for muscular work in young men. *Research Quarterly, 14*:31-36, March, 1943.

[2] CARLSON, H. C.: Fatigue curve test. *Research Quarterly, 16*: 169-175, October, 1945.

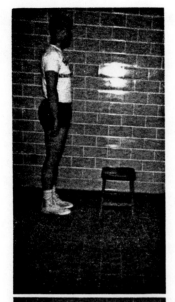

Brouha step test. Starting position.

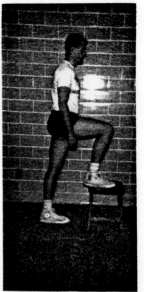

Step down with the right foot.

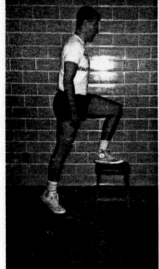

Step up with the left foot.

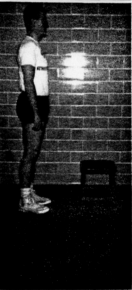

Step down with the left foot.

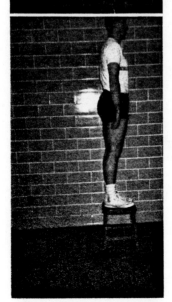

Step up with the right foot.

STRENGTH EXERCISE

In the off-season, pre-season and regular season, all players should do some strength exercises to maintain their strength and to stay "stretched out." Thirty-six second pull-ups, push-ups and shoulder dips are excellent exercises to maintain your shoulder and arm strength.

Spring training is a time to perfect your skills and learn new ones. Players should not waste the whole spring training trying to lose the weight they gained over the winter and attempting to regain their former strength and cardiovascular condition. They should report to spring training ready to play ball. Little leaguers, high school, college and university players should be ready to play the first day of practice.

High school and college seasons are short, due to cold spring weather in the northern schools and school being out in late May or early June. Do your strength exercises often in the off-season and pre-season. During the regular season, one thirty-six second pull-up, push-up and shoulder dip will maintain your strength.

Pull-ups, push-ups and shoulder dips are a controversial subject for baseball players. Many old-time baseball coaches say, "Do not do any exercise with the arm and shoulder, you will hurt your arm." Yet these same men want their players to sprint and exercise the rest of the body. It is better for pitchers to just hang from a bar to stretch the arms and shoulders instead of doing pull-ups. All other players do pull-ups.

Baseball players need strength in their arms, shoulders, wrists, fingers and the whole body. Years ago, most of our baseball players were farm boys who did many types of strength work with their hands, arms, shoulders and whole body in their daily work. Today, however, even farm boys are weaker because of mechanization.

It takes months and years of strenuous resistive exercise to add inches of girth to muscles. Baseball players need strong, long and loose muscles. Pull-ups, push-ups and shoulder dips will give the baseball player strength, and the stretching at the end of pull-ups and push-ups will keep their muscles stretched out. The strong, loose players have very few injuries because they strengthen and stretch all the muscles in the body.

Pull-ups

A number of great professional baseball players do pull-ups and push-ups daily throughout the year to maintain and increase shoulder and hand strength. Put up a chinning bar outside or inside your home so you can do pull-ups daily throughout the off-season.

Pull-ups may be done isometrically by holding for six seconds at different points throughout the pull-up. Each complete pull-up takes thirty-six seconds. To add more resistance, weights may be applied by wearing a weighted vest or a weighted belt around the waist.

Pull-ups should be done with different grips—the palms away from the body and the palms facing the body. Thirty-six second pull-ups are done in the following manner: (a) pull-up flexing the elbows about 15 degrees and hold for six seconds; (b) pull-up flexing the elbows to 90 degrees and hold for six seconds; (c) pull-up looking over the bar and hold for six seconds; (d) lower slowly to 90 degrees of elbow flexion and hold for six seconds; (e) lower slowly to 15 degrees of elbow flexion and hold for six seconds; (f) lower to complete elbow extension and hold stretching for six seconds.

Do at least three pull-ups daily for thirty-six seconds in the off-season and pre-season and one pull-up daily during the regular season. Be sure to use the different hand grips while holding the bar. See the pictures on page 19.

Pull-up flexing the elbows 15 degrees.

Lower to 90 degrees of elbow flexion.

Pull-up flexing the elbows 90 degrees.

Lower to 15 degrees of elbow flexion.

Chin over the bar.

Lower to complete extension—stretch.

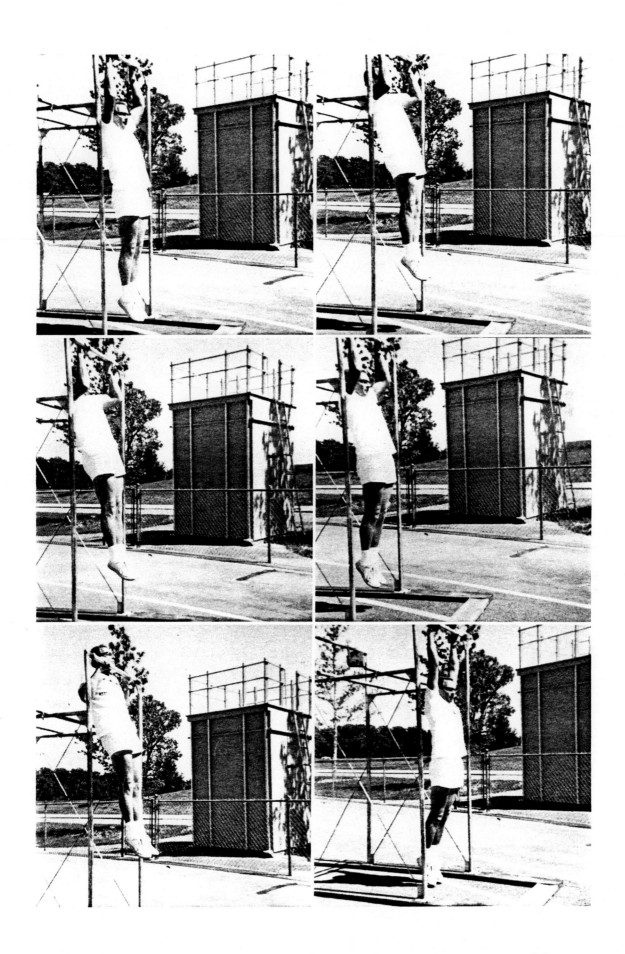

Push-ups

Baseball players do push-ups to strengthen the fingers, wrists, arms and chest. Push-ups may be done several ways: with your hands close together forming a triangle with your fingers and thumbs under your chest; with your hands wide outside your shoulders; or with your hands directly under the shoulders. They may also be done with your hands on two chairs, lowering the body between the chairs to get a good stretch across the chest. See the pictures below.

Hands on the chairs.

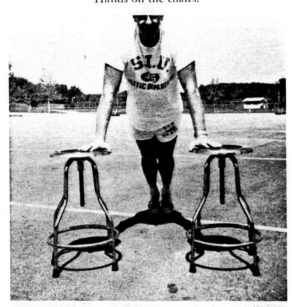

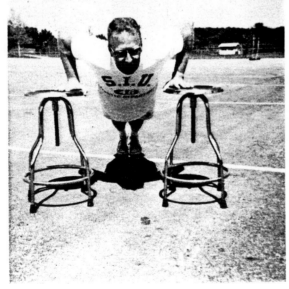

Lower the body between the chairs—stretch.

Do ten to fifteen push-ups daily in the off-season and pre-season, slowly pushing up and down. Do one or two daily during the regular season to maintain your strength. More resistance may be added by putting your feet up on a chair with your hands on the floor. You may also do thirty-six second isometric push-ups as you do in pull-ups and shoulder dips. Many baseball players do their push-ups on their finger tips to strengthen the fingers.

Shoulder Dips

Shoulder dips are another method to help develop your shoulders and arm strength. Dips may be done between the backs of two sturdy chairs or on your parallel bars outside or in your basement.

The thirty-six second shoulder dip is one of the better methods for developing arm and shoulder strength. Thirty-six second isometric shoulder dips are done in the following manner: (a) with the elbows completely extended, lower the body flexing the elbows about 15 degrees and hold for six seconds; (b) slowly lower the body flexing the elbows to 90 degrees and hold for six seconds; (c) lower the body to complete elbow flexion and hold for six seconds; (d) push the body up to 90 degrees of elbow flexion and hold for six seconds; (e) push the body up to 15 degrees of elbow flexion and hold for six seconds; (f) push the body as far as possible, completely extending the elbows and hold for six seconds.

Do at least three shoulder dips daily for thirty-six seconds in the off-season and pre-season and one shoulder dip daily during the regular season to maintain your strength.

WARM-UP EXERCISES

All baseball players should stretch and do warm-up exercises before any activity; they should sprint to get the muscles ready for the activity. How much warm-up you do will depend on the weather, your age, old injuries, your present state of physical fitness and many more variables. Warming-up is an individual problem, but be sure you are warm and loose in order to avoid injury. See pages 30-49.

STRETCHING EXERCISES USING SHOWER ROOM PROCEDURE

1. Heel Cord Stretch

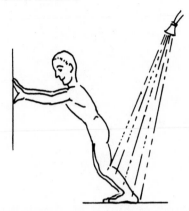

   a. Hold six seconds—relax—repeat three to six times.

2. Hamstring Stretch

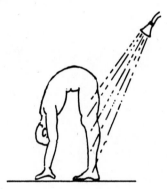

   a. Hold six seconds—relax—repeat three to six times.

3. Back Stretch

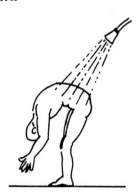

   a. Hold six seconds—relax—repeat three to six times.

4. Back and Shoulder Stretch (Hang by Hands)

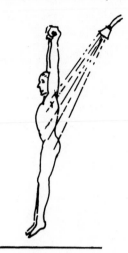

   a. Tilt pelvis forward and backward.
   b. Hold six seconds each way—relax—repeat three to six times.

5. Back and Side Stretch (Both Sides)

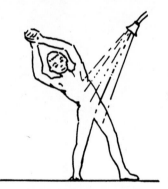

   a. Hold six seconds—relax—repeat three to six times.
   b. Stretch both sides.

6. Chest and Shoulder Stretch

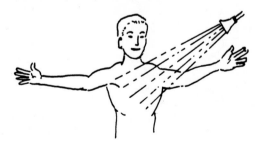

   a. Hold six seconds—relax—repeat three to six times.

7. Chest and Shoulder Stretch Overhead

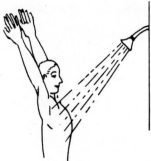

a. Hold six seconds—relax—repeat three to six times.

8. Shoulder Rotators Stretch (Internal and External Rotators)

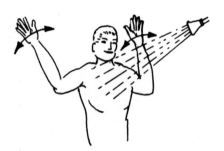

a. Rotate shoulders outward—hold six seconds—relax—repeat three to six times.

b. Rotate shoulders inward—hold six seconds—relax—repeat three to six times.

c. Also turn back to shower.

9. Wrist Stretch (Flexing and Extending)

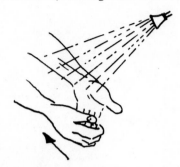

a. Stretch wrist down—hold six seconds—relax—repeat three to six times.

b. Stretch wrist back—hold six seconds—relax—repeat three to six times.

c. Stretch both wrists.

10. Biceps Stretch

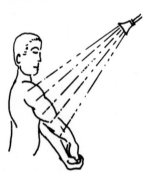

a. Hold elbow straight—pull back on wrist pushing elbow forward.

b. Hold six seconds—relax—repeat three to six times.

c. Stretch both arms.

ISOMETRIC EXERCISE PROCEDURE

1. One person does the exercise. A partner provides the resistance. Change positions. Your partner does the exercise while you resist. In the beginning do not try to exert full effort.
2. Each man repeats the exercise three times, resisting six seconds each time.
3. Push or pull as hard as possible for six seconds, relax six seconds, push six seconds, relax six seconds, push six seconds, relax.
4. There should be little or no movement through a range of motion during the isometric exercise.
5. When resisting, do not push so hard that your partner cannot maintain the correct angle.
6. When resisting, be sure you make your partner push as hard as he can while maintaining the correct angle.
7. You should not experience pain during the exercise. Should you have any pain, ease off and push as hard as you can without pain. As strength increases the pain will leave. If pain continues, consult your physician before resuming any exercise.
8. Never push so hard that you feel like you may black out when pushing or pulling. An individual can gain in strength pushing or pulling at 50 per cent to 70 per cent of his best effort.
9. Begin each contraction slowly and ease off the contraction slowly at the end of the six-second contraction.
10. Exercise at least three different positions through a complete range of motion to strengthen the entire muscle—15 degrees, 45 degrees and 90 degrees.

STRETCHING EXERCISE PROCEDURE

1. Stretching exercises should be done daily along with isometric exercises.
2. When there is tightness in any area, in order to gain in range of motion, it is better to stretch after some type of heat has been applied to the area being stretched. For example, there may be tightness in the back and back of the legs. This tightness limits the length of a stride in running and makes it difficult to flex from the waist. Bend over in the shower and heat the area well. Then bend over slowly and stretch, holding the position for six seconds. Do not bob up and down to force a stretch, as many individuals do—this may cause an injury by overstretching tight muscles. Follow the stretching procedure under number 4 below.
3. Where extreme tightness exists, it is best to stretch daily in the shower room after applying a hot shower to heat the area, increase the circulation and relax the tight muscles.
4. Stretching is done best in the following manner: (1) allow hot water to heat the part in the shower; (b) stretch in the same method used in exercising; (c) stretch as far as you can until you feel a little pain; (d) hold this position for six seconds, relax six seconds, try to go a little farther again and hold six seconds, relax six seconds, try to go a little farther again and hold for six seconds, relax. See pictures on pages 21 and 22.
5. Repeat the same procedure in stretching all tight areas of the body. Repeat daily until you gain complete range, if possible.

OFF-SEASON CONDITIONING

Stretching Exercises

Chest and Shoulder Stretch

1. Standing
   a. Hold a broomstick (42-45 in.) in front of the body in the palms of the hands.
   b. Keep the elbows straight.
   c. Lift the broomstick forward and over the head slowly.
   d. Stretch for six seconds and slowly return; relax.
   e. Repeat three times, stretching a little farther each time.

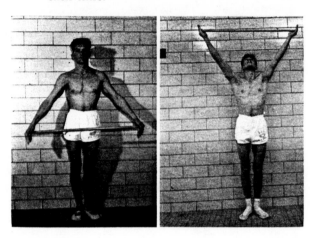

2. Standing
   a. Hold a broomstick out to the side of the body.
   b. Keep the elbow straight on the arm overhead.
   c. Push the broomstick up to the side slowly.
   d. Stretch for six seconds and slowly push the broomstick up to the other side. Stretch for six seconds.
   e. Repeat three times, stretching a little farther each time.

3. Standing
   a. Hold a broomstick in front of the body.
   b. Push the broomstick up in front of the body on one side.
   c. Keep the elbow straight on the arm overhead.
   d. Stretch for six seconds and return to the front of the body.
   e. Push the broomstick up in front of the body to the other side.
   f. Repeat three times, stretching a little farther each time.

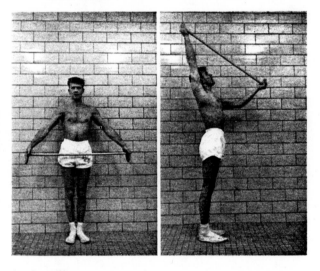

4. Standing
   a. Hold a broomstick behind the body.
   b. Keep the elbows straight.

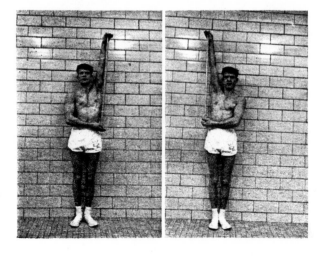

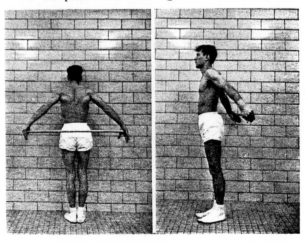

c. Push the broomstick backward as high as possible.

d. Keep the body straight. Do not bend forward.

e. Stretch for six seconds and return to the starting position.

f. Repeat three times, stretching a little farther each time.

5. Standing

a. Hold a broomstick behind the body.

b. Push the broomstick up to the side.

c. Keep the elbow straight on the overhead arm.

d. Stretch for six seconds, and return to the starting position.

e. Push the broomstick up to the other side.

f. Stretch for six seconds and return; relax.

g. Repeat three times, stretching a little farther each time.

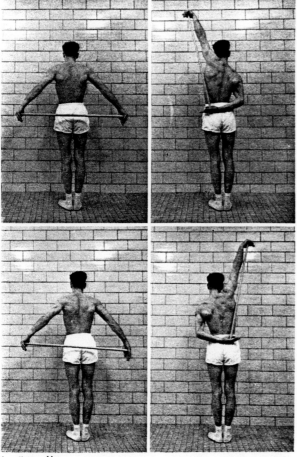

6. Standing

a. Hold a broomstick overhead in the palms of the hands.

b. Keep the elbows straight. The feet are about 18 inches apart.

c. Bend sideward as far as possible, keeping the elbows straight.

d. Stretch for six seconds and return to the starting position.

e. Bend sideward as far as possible to the other side.

f. Stretch for six seconds and return to the starting position.

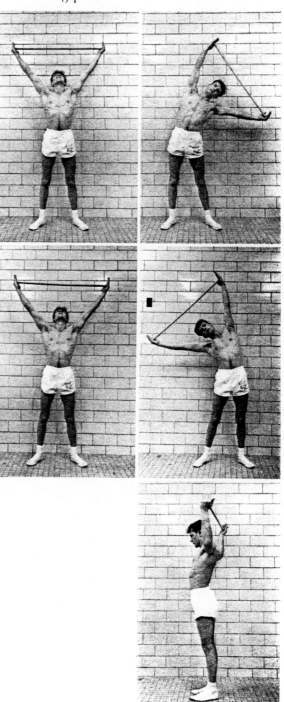

g. Repeat three times, stretching a little farther
    each time.
7. Standing
    a. Hold a broomstick overhead in the palms of
        the hands.
    b. The shoulders are raised to 90 degrees, and
        the elbows are bent to 90 degrees.
    c. Rotate the arms backward as far as possible.
    d. Stretch for six seconds and return to the
        starting position.
    e. Repeat three times, stretching a little farther
        each time. See pictures on page 25.

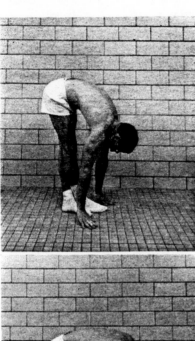

Back of the Leg Stretch (Hamstrings)

1. Standing
    a. Cross one leg in front of the other leg. The feet are close
        together.
    b. Hold the rear leg back with the front leg.
    c. Keep both knees straight.
    d. Bend over and touch the floor beside the feet.
    e. Stretch for six seconds and return.
    f. Place the other leg in front.
    g. Stretch for six seconds and return.
    h. Repeat three times with each leg forward, stretching a
        little farther each time.

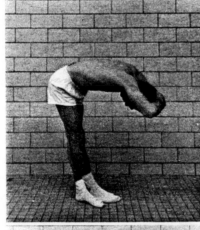

2. Standing
    a. Cross one leg in front of the other leg. The feet are close
        together.
    b. Bend the elbows and fold the arms in front of the body
        up near the head.
    c. Bend over as far as possible and stretch out with the
        elbows.
    d. Stretch for six seconds and return.
    e. Repeat three times, bending and stretching a little farther
        each time.
    f. Place the other leg in front.
    g. Stretch for six seconds and return.
    h. Repeat three times, bending and stretching a little farther
        each time.

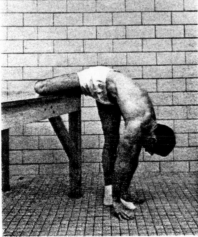

3. Standing
    a. Raise one leg on a table or a hurdle with the knee bent.
    b. Bend over and try to touch the floor beside the foot.
    c. Keep the leg and knee straight.
    d. Stretch for six seconds and return.
    e. Raise the other leg on the table.
    f. Bend over and try to touch the floor beside the foot.
    g. Stretch for six seconds and return. Try to put the palms
        flat on the floor.
    h. Repeat three times with each leg, stretching a little farther
        each time.

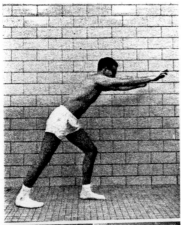

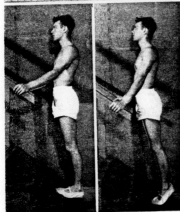

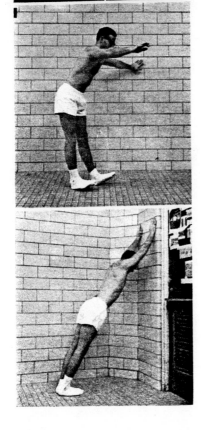

Heel Cord Stretch

1. Standing
   a. Step forward with the left leg.
   b. Keep the right leg back with the knee held straight.
   c. Bend the left knee and bring the body forward, keeping both feet pointing straight ahead.
   d. Keep the right heel on the floor and stretch the right heel cord for six seconds.
   e. Step forward with the right leg.
   f. Keep the left heel on the floor and stretch the left heel cord for six seconds.
   g. Repeat three times with each leg, stretching a little farther each time.

2. Standing on the stairs
   a. Stand with the balls of the feet on the edge of the stairs.
   b. Rise on the toes as high as possible, holding for six seconds.
   c. Drop down off the edge of the stairs stretching the heel cords for six seconds.
   d. Rise up and down three times, stretching a little farther each time.

3. Standing
   a. Walk on the heels with the ball of the foot off the ground.
   b. Stretch the foot up hard, walking at least 30 yds — relax.
   c. Repeat three times, stretching a little farther each time.

4. Standing
   a. Place the hands against the wall at shoulder height.
   b. Keep the heels on the floor.
   c. Move backward until you feel a good stretch on the heel cords.
   d. Stretch the heel cords for six seconds.
   e. Repeat three times, stretching a little farther each time.

Wrist Stretching and Strengthening

1. Standing
   a. Raise the left arm straight out in front of the body.
   b. Bend the left wrist down with the palm of the hand forward.
   c. Grasp the left palm with the right hand stretching the wrist down and back for six seconds.
   d. Repeat three times with each wrist, stretching a little farther each time.
   e. Turn the hand over and stretch the wrist the other way.
   f. Repeat three times with each wrist, stretching a little farther each time.

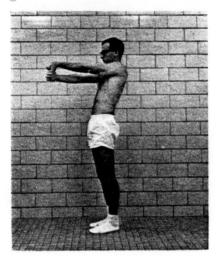

2. Standing (Weighted bat exercises)
   a. Hold a weighted bar in front of the body.
   b. Keep the elbow straight with the weight pointing toward the floor.
   c. Lift the weight up slowly taking six seconds to raise.

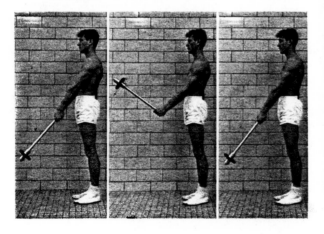

   d. Slowly lower the weight taking six seconds to lower to the starting position.
   e. Repeat three times with each wrist.
   f. Add more weight when three repetitions become easy.

3. Standing
   a. Hold a weighted bar behind the body.
   b. Keep the elbow straight with the weight pointing toward the floor.
   c. Lift the weight up slowly taking six seconds to raise.
   d. Slowly lower the weight taking six seconds to lower to the starting position.
   e. Repeat three times with each wrist.
   f. Add more weight when three repetitions become easy.

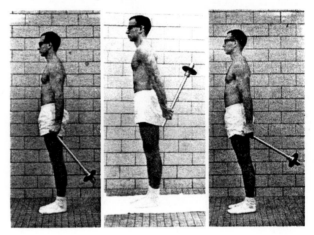

4. Standing
   a. Hold a weighted bar in front of the body with the elbow straight.

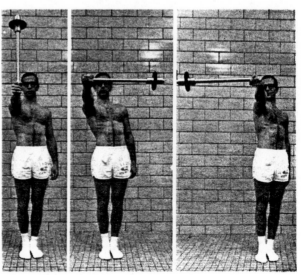

b. Raise the arm up straight in front of the body to shoulder height.

c. Slowly pronate (turn) the hand lowering the weight to the inside taking three seconds to lower. Keep the elbow straight.

d. Slowly return to the starting position taking three seconds to return.

e. Slowly supinate (turn) the hand lowering the weight to the outside taking three seconds to lower and three seconds to return.

f. Repeat three times with each wrist.

g. Add more weight when three repetitions become easy.

h. Do exercises 1, 2, 3, and 4 with weighted bat daily. See page 7.

5. Standing
    a. Hold a bar out in front of the body with a rope and a weight tied to the end.
    b. Slowly roll the weight up on the bar. Keep the elbows straight.
    c. Reach under the bar as far as possible and roll the wrist over the top.
    d. Slowly roll the weight down to the starting position.
    e. Repeat three times rolling the weight up and down.
    f. Five lbs is a good starting weight.
    g. Add more weight when three repetitions become easy.

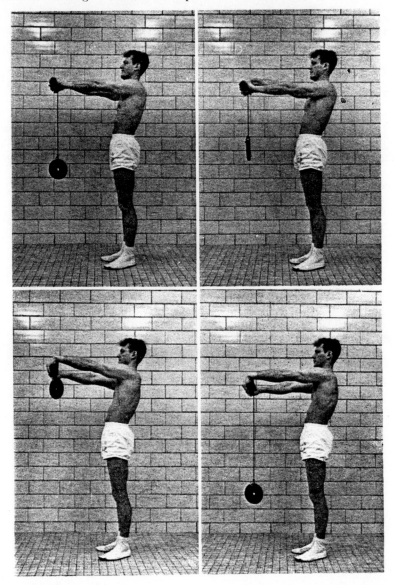

WARM-UP EXERCISES

1. Side Straddle Hop Bend

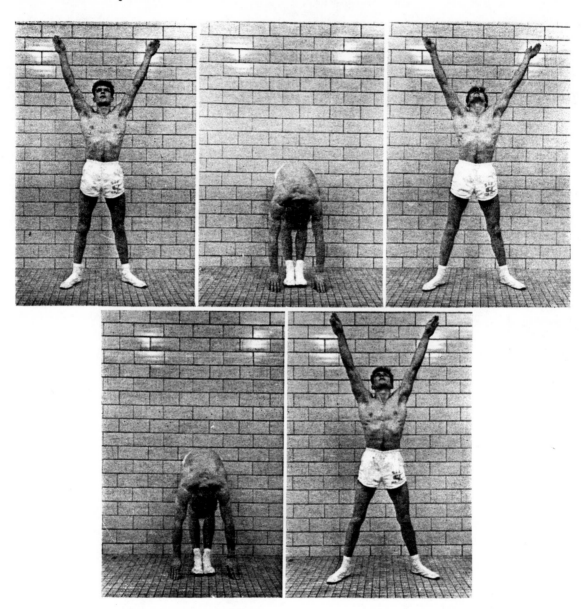

2. Trunk Rotation—Standing with a Broomstick in Elbows Behind Back

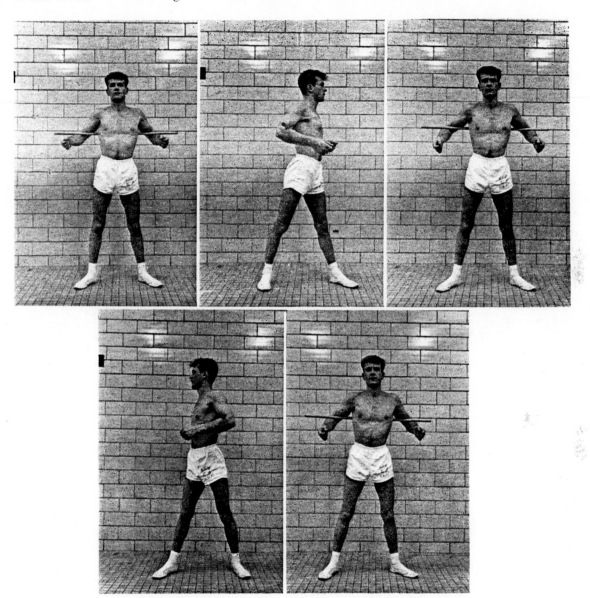

3.   Alternate Toe Touch

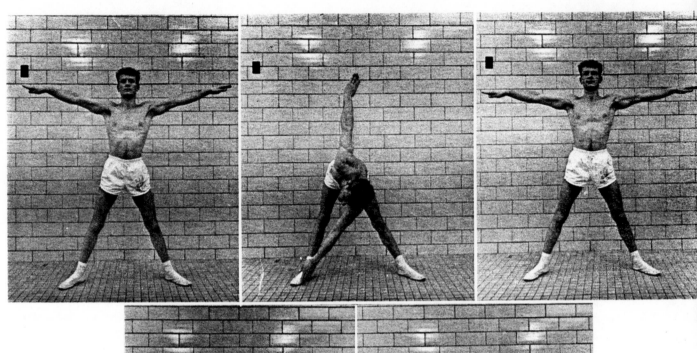

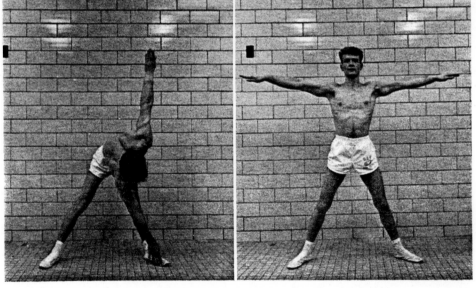

4. Side Bender

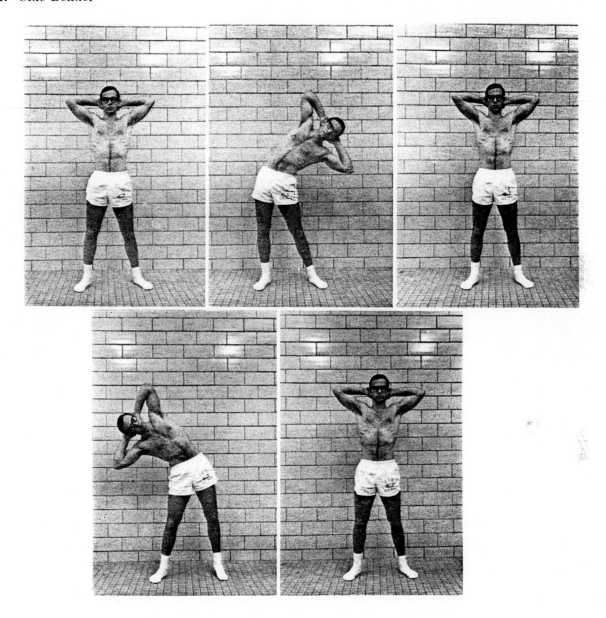

5. Trunk Rotation

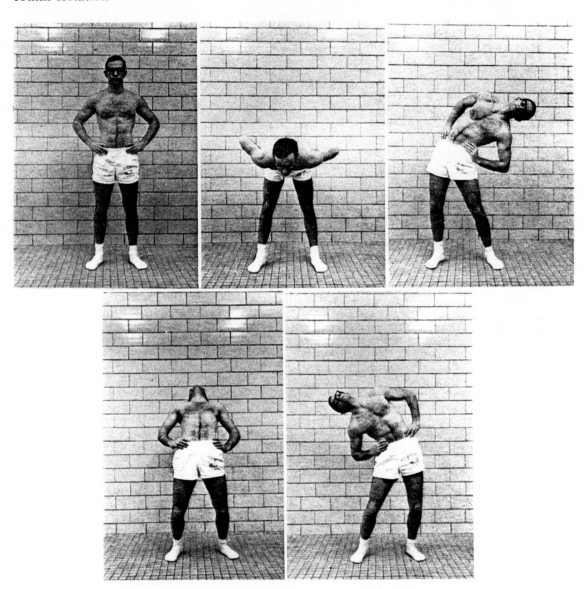

6. Burpee with a Push-up

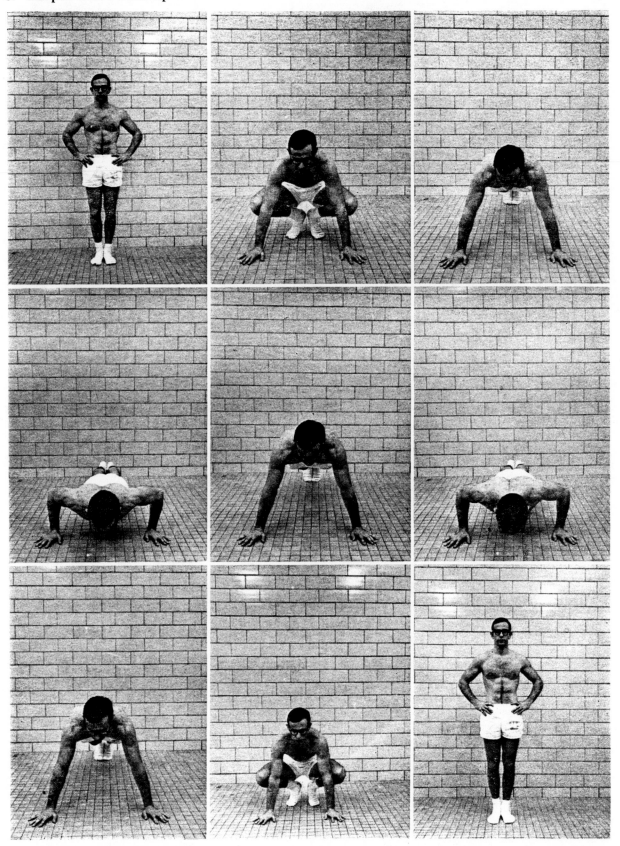

7. Leg Extension Sideward from a Squat Position

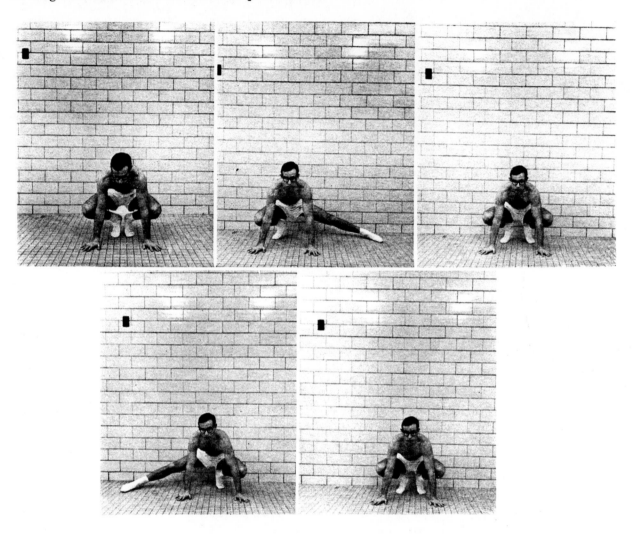

8. Sit-up with a Partner

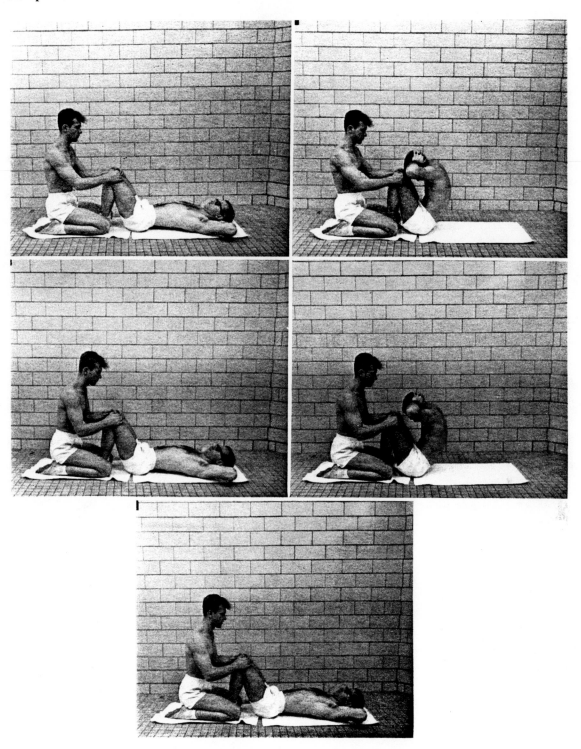

9. Alternate Leg Lift (Hamstring Stretch)

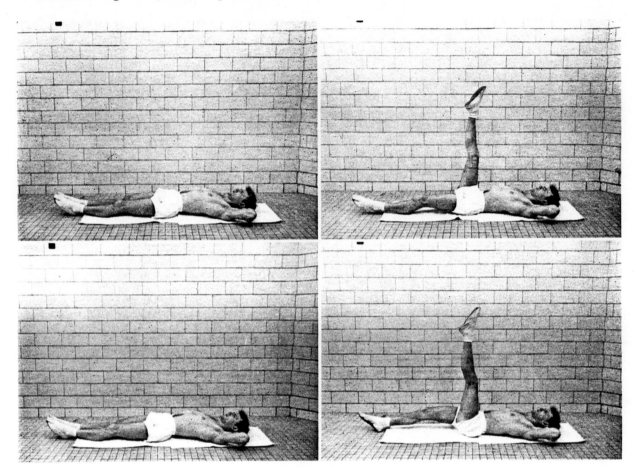

10.   Alternate Knee to Chest

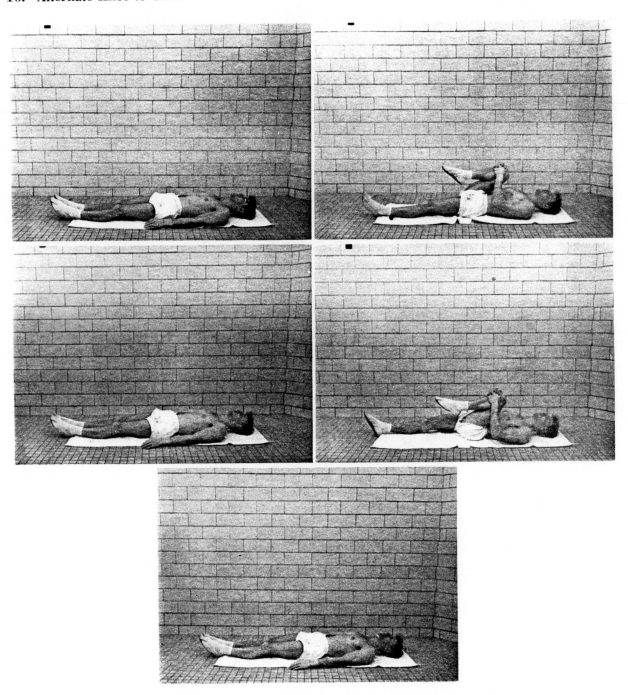

11. Double Knee to Chest

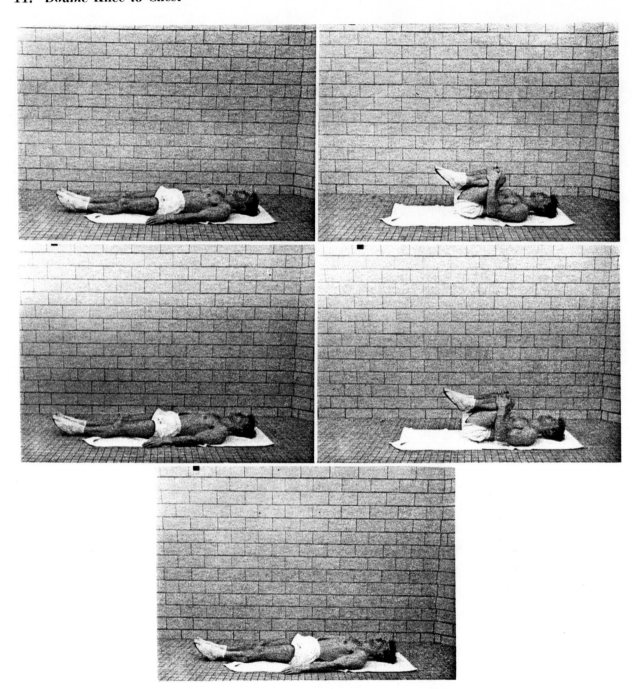

12. Rowing Exercise

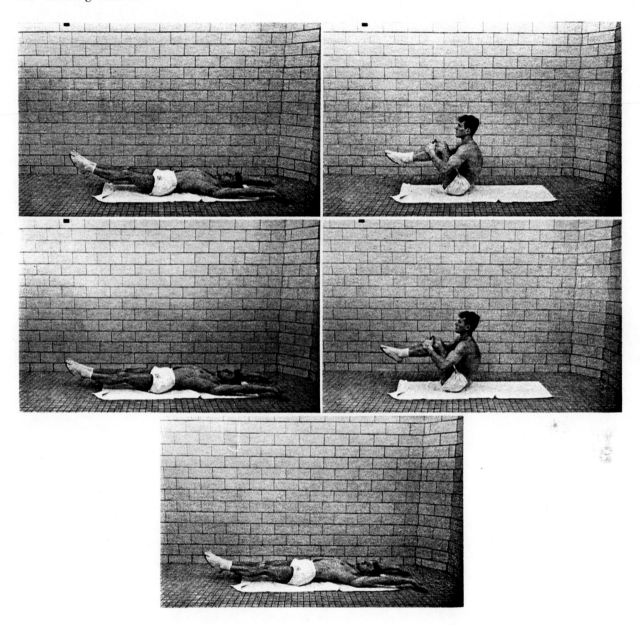

13. Hip Raiser

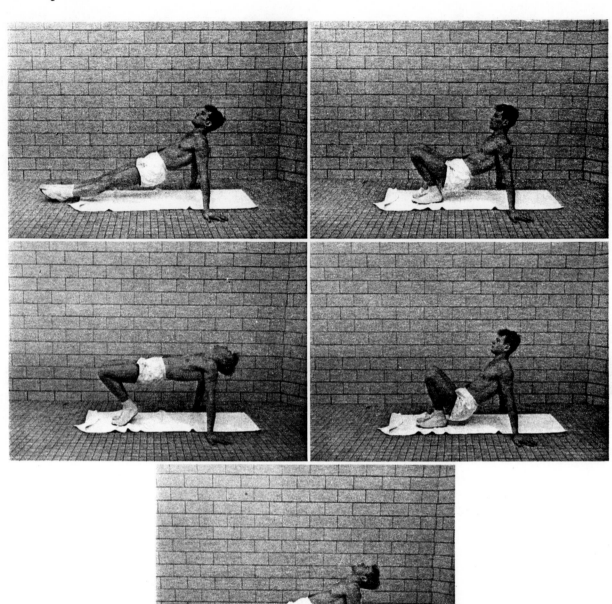

14. Back Shuffler from Back Leaning Rest Position

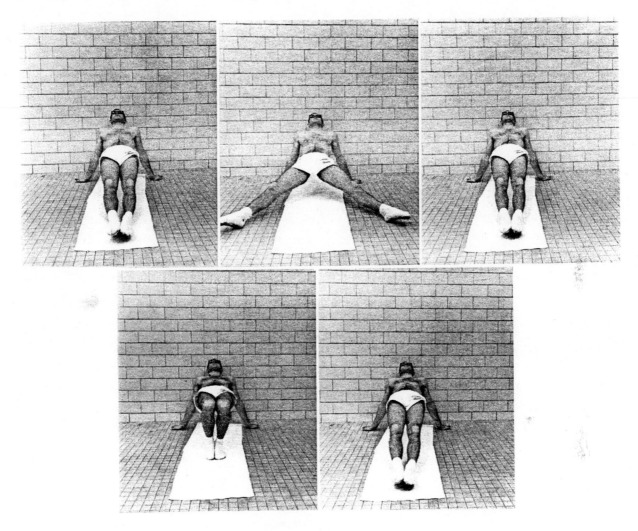

15. Leg Kick from Back Leaning Rest Position—Feet 18 in. Apart

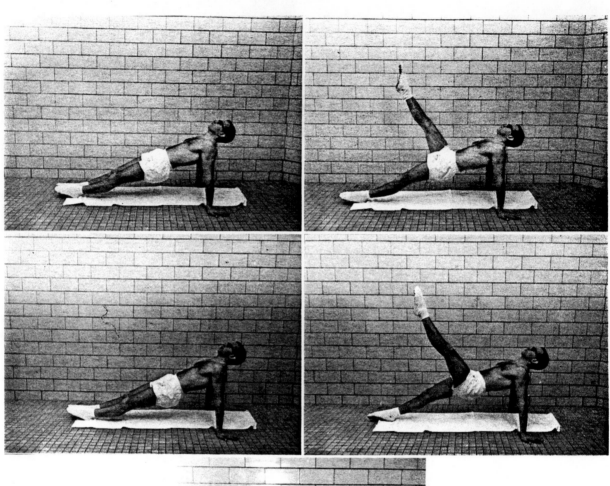

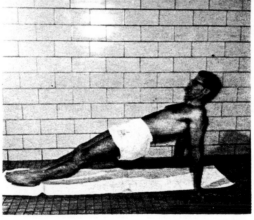

16. Horizontal Running (Full Squat—Hands on the Ground)

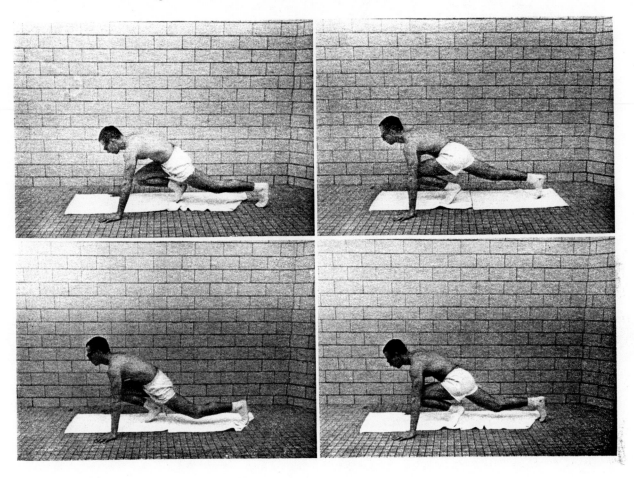

17. Push-ups

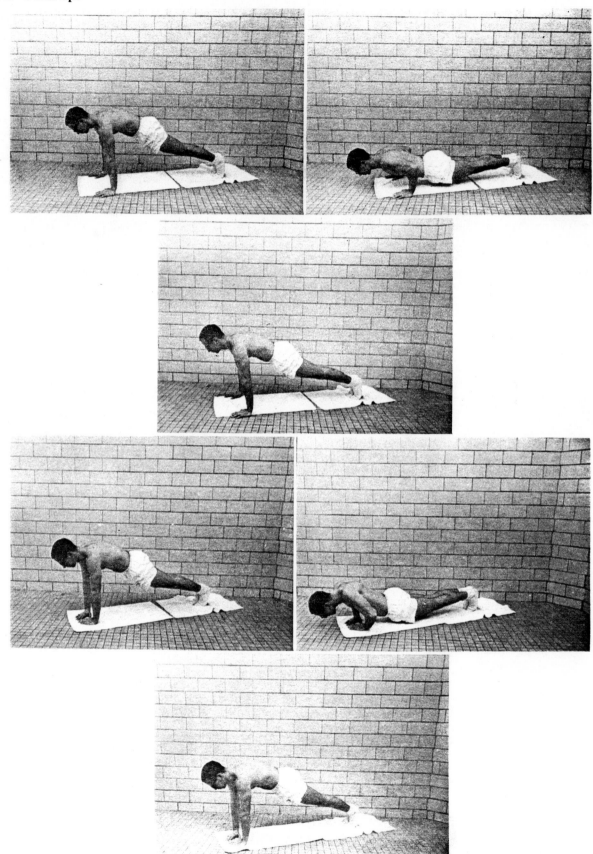

18. Opposite Leg and Arm Raiser

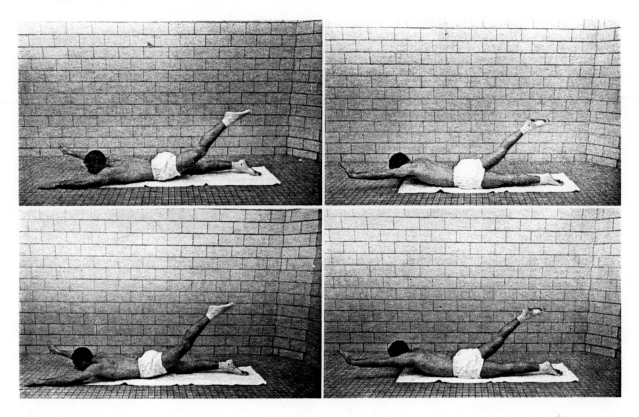

19. Leg Crossover from Back Lying Position

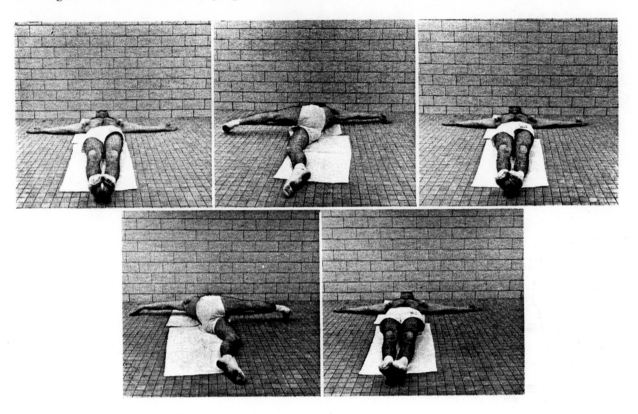

20. Leg Lift Side Lying—Exercise Both Legs

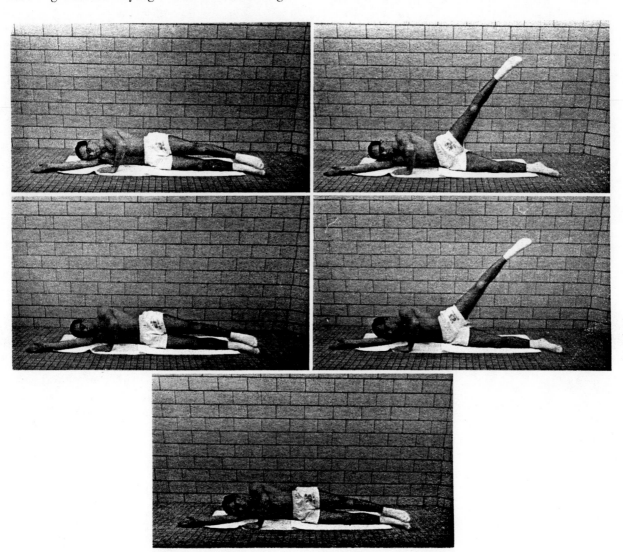

STRENGTHEN ALL WEAK AREAS

All weak areas should be strengthened in the off-season and pre-season conditioning programs. Every athlete has some area in the body that is weak and needs strengthening exercise. Weakness may be due to having some area in the body in which a player has never developed any strength. We know from research that any area that has been injured must be restrengthened before every season and kept strengthened by daily resistive exercise throughout the season.

When we have a muscle tear or a ligament sprain, the body repairs this injury with scar tissue. Scar tissue never functions like normal tissue. It never has the same blood supply; it is not elastic as it was originally; it does not have the same sensory nerve supply. We can redevelop the strength in this injured area, but if we do not do some resistive exercise daily to keep it strong throughout the season, the strength will drop off. Through disuse or sometimes even normal activity in baseball games, we may lose 20 to 50 lbs. of strength as the season goes on. Without resistive exercise we usually reinjure the weak area or injure another area protecting those weak muscles.

Each individual player must find out how much resistive exercise he needs to keep his weak area strong. Every injury is different, so perhaps you may find you need to do resistive exercise only twice a week to stay strong. Others may have to exercise daily to stay strong. Find out how much exercise you need to keep your weak ankle, leg, back, shoulder or arm strong, and keep exercising it.

After your strengthening exercises, stretching and cardiovascular exercise, you should always swing your favorite bat. Your bat should always feel light in your hands. Professional baseball players should all have enough extra strength to be able to swing a 40- to 50-oz. bat, even though they prefer a 33- to 35-oz. bat. With enough strength to swing a 40-oz. bat, your regular bat will always feel light. Little league, high school and college baseball players should all have strong hands, arms and shoulders, so that the bat they like feels light in their hands.

Players are strong and in good physical condition when the season begins, but many get weaker as the season goes along. We see this every season. A player begins the season using a 35-oz. bat. In two months he says he cannot get the 35-oz. bat around and changes to a 33-oz. bat. This may be due to many things, such as timing, overstriding, a hitch in his swing, taking his eye off the ball or loss of strength, or it may be all psychological.

Questioning many players, one finds that they say they do not feel strong enough to swing their regular 35-oz. bats. For this reason they should exercise with a weighted bat, a medi exercise ball and other resistive exercise throughout the season to maintain and perhaps even increase their strength in the weak area. See pages 7 and 8.

In the off-season and pre-season, you should take fifty to one hundred swings daily with your regular, favorite model bat. This will get your hands tough and ready for the season. To protect your hands, you may purchase a pair of golf gloves. A number of baseball players use golf gloves during the season for a better grip on the bat and also to protect the hands. Coaches also use the golf gloves to protect the hands when using the fungo bat so often during the season.

To improve your swing in the off-season or pre-season, it is advisable to take your swings in front of a mirror. This way you can be sure your swing is level, and you will be hitting the ball in front of the plate. Using a batting tee and hitting balls into a screen will also help the hitter who is weak on hitting low balls or high balls or who has any other weakness. You can easily make your own batting tee and screen. Be sure to strengthen all of your weak areas.

ISOMETRIC EXERCISE

Isometric exercise is one of the best and quickest methods for baseball players to increase their strength. Find a partner and work the weak areas daily using isometric exercise for thirty minutes. In the off-season, every other day or three days a week may be enough. Six weeks before spring training or practice begins, you should step up your stretching, strength and cardiovascular exercise program. Work five to seven days a week for at least one hour a day.

Before beginning your isometric exercise always spend at least ten minutes doing stretching and warm-up exercises. Choose the exercises carefully to strengthen your weak areas and the areas of the body that are most essential for baseball. In a thirty- to forty-minute period with a two-man isometric program, you can work all the muscles in the body.

Follow the exercises closely to be sure they are done correctly in order to achieve the desired results.

Neck Exercises

After engaging in selected stretching and warm-up exercises, we shall begin the two-man isometric exercises at the neck and work downward. Each exercise is given to exercise the prime movers, the major muscles that initiate the action in any movement. Follow the exercises closely to be sure they are done correctly in order to achieve the desired results. See isometric exercise procedure on page 23.

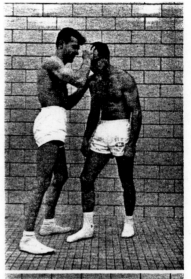

1. Neck Flexion

   a. Bring your chin towards your chest.

   b. Your partner attempts to push your head back, resisting for six seconds with his palm on your forehead.

   c. Your partner does the same exercise bringing his head towards his chest.

   d. Resist for six seconds with your palm on his forehead.

   e. Each man repeats the exercise three times for a total of eighteen seconds exercise for each man.

2. Neck Extension

   a. Push your head back as far as possible.

   b. Your partner attempts to push your head forward, resisting for six seconds with his palm on the back of your head.

   c. Your partner does the same exercise pushing his head back as far as possible.

   d. Resist for six seconds with your palm on the back of his head.

   e. Each man repeats the exercise three times for a total of eighteen seconds exercise for each man.

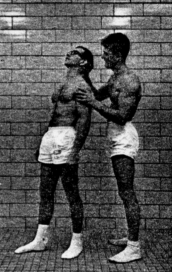

3. Neck Lateral Flexion

   a. Push your head to the side, bringing your ear toward your shoulder.

   b. Your partner attempts to push your head back to a straight position, resisting for six seconds with his palm on the side of your head.

   c. Your partner does the same exercise pushing his head to the side bringing his ear towards his shoulder.

   d. Resist for six seconds with your palm on the side of his head.

   e. Repeat the exercise pushing your head toward the other shoulder.

   f. Each man repeats the exercise three times on each side for a total of thirty-six seconds of exercise for each man.

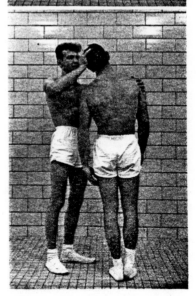

Shoulder and Arm Exercises

1. Shoulder Flexion (Lift Arms Forward)

a. Raise the arms forward to 90 degrees with the elbows straight and the palms down. Keep your stomach muscles tight and your back straight.

b. Your partner attempts to push your arms down toward the floor, resisting for six seconds with his palms on the back of your hand and wrist.

c. Your partner does the same exercise bringing his arms forward to 90 degrees. Be sure not to lean backward. Keep your stomach muscles tight.

d. Resist for six seconds with your palm on the back of his hand and wrist.

e. Each man repeats the exercise three times.

f. Exercise at three different positions through a complete range of motion in shoulder flexion—15 degrees, 45 degrees and at 90 degrees as shown in the picture.

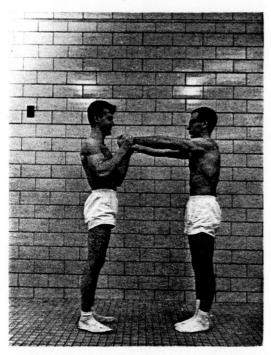

2. Shoulder Abduction (Lift Arms Sideward)

a. Raise the arms sideward to 90 degrees with the elbows straight and the palms down. Keep your stomach muscles tight and your back straight.

b. Your partner attempts to push your arms down toward the floor, resisting for six sec-

onds with his palms on the back of your hand and wrist.

c. Your partner does the same exercise raising his arms sideward to 90 degrees. Be sure not to lean backward. Keep your stomach muscles tight.

d. Resist for six seconds with your palm on the back of his hand and wrist.

e. Each man repeats the exercise three times.

f. Exercise at three different positions through a complete range of motion in shoulder abduction—15 degrees, 45 degrees and at 90 degrees as shown in the picture.

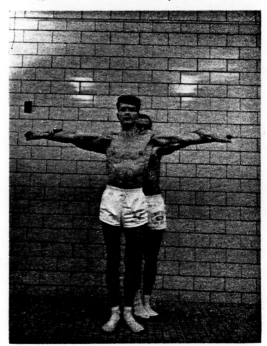

3. Shoulder Horizontal Extension (Push Arms Backward)

a. With your back to your partner, raise the arms to 90 degrees, palms down. Push the arms backward, pinching the shoulder blades together. Keep the arms raised to 90 degrees and the stomach muscles tight.

b. Your partner attempts to push your arms forward, resisting for six seconds with his palms on the side of your hand and wrist.

c. Your partner does the same exercise pushing his arms backward, pinching his shoulder blades together. Be sure to keep the elbows straight, arms raised to 90 degrees and the stomach muscles tight.

d. Brace yourself with one foot forward, and do

not lean backward while exercising.

e. Resist for six seconds with your palms on the side of his hand and wrist.

f. Each man repeats the exercise three times.

g. Exercise at three different positions through a complete range of motion in shoulder horizontal extension—15 degrees, arms in front of the body, 45 degrees and at 90 degrees as shown in the picture.

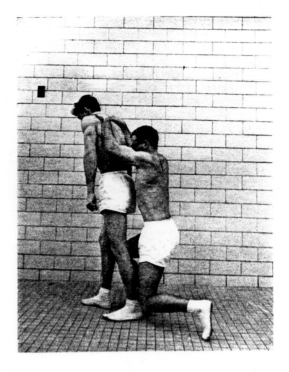

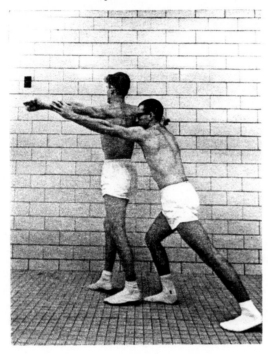

NOTE:

1. All shoulder exercises except numbers 4, 7 and 8 can be done sitting in a chair facing your partner.

2. When working with two people or in small groups, better stabilization can be maintained while sitting in a chair.

3. When working with athletic teams or large

4. Shoulder Shrug

a. With your back to your partner, raise your shoulders as high as possible, bringing your shoulders toward your ears with your elbows bent.

b. Your partner hangs all of his body weight on your shoulders and attempts to pull your shoulders down, resisting for six seconds.

c. Your partner does the same exercise, hanging his body weight on your shoulders. You may have to lean forward a little to keep your balance.

d. Resist for six seconds with your body weight hanging on his shoulders.

e. Each man repeats the exercise three times.

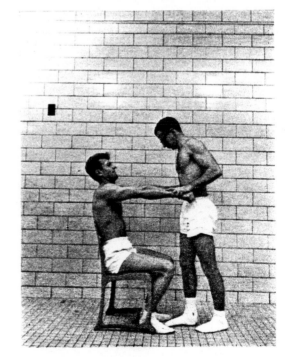

groups, the exercises may be done standing, with special emphasis on keeping the abdominal muscles tight and standing up straight.

4. Exercise at three different positions through a complete range of motion—15 degrees, 45 degrees and at 90 degrees as shown in the pictures.

5. Shoulder Elevation Sideward

a. Raise the arms sideward and backward to an overhead position to about 135 degrees, keeping the elbows straight and the palms facing forward.

b. Your partner attempts to pull your arms downward toward the floor, resisting for six seconds with his palms on the thumb and wrist.

c. Your partner does the same exercise raising his arms sideward and backward to an overhead position to about 135 degrees. Keep your elbows straight and do not lean backward.

d. Resist for six seconds with your palms on the thumb and wrist.

e. Each man repeats the exercise three times.

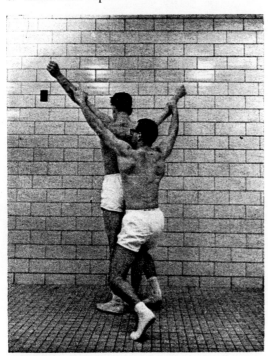

6. Shoulder External Rotation

a. Raise the arms sideward to 90 degrees, and bend the elbows to 90 degrees with the palms forward.

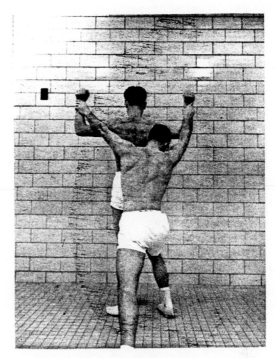

b. Rotate your shoulders outward.

c. Your partner attempts to rotate your shoulders forward by grasping your wrists, resisting for six seconds.

d. Your partner does the same exercise raising his arms sideward to 90 degrees and bending his elbows to 90 degrees. Keep your stomach muscles tight.

e. Resist for six seconds by grasping his wrists and atempting to rotate his shoulders internally.

f. Each man repeats the exercise three times.

g. Exercise at three different positions through a complete range of motion in shoulder external rotation—45 degrees, 90 degrees, as shown in the picture and at complete external rotation.

7. Shoulder Internal Rotation

a. Raise the arms sideward to 90 degrees and bend the elbows to 90 degrees with the palms forward.

b. Rotate your shoulders internally. Keep your stomach muscles tight.

c. Your partner attempts to push your shoulders externally by grasping your wrists, resisting for six seconds.

d. Your partner does the same exercise raising his arms sideward to 90 degrees and bending his elbows to 90 degrees. Keep your stomach muscles tight.

e. Resist for six seconds by grasping his wrists and attempting to rotate his shoulders externally.

f. Each man repeats the exercise three times.

g. Exercise at three different positions through a complete range of motion in shoulder internal rotation—complete external rotation, 90 degrees, as shown in the picture, and at 45 degrees.

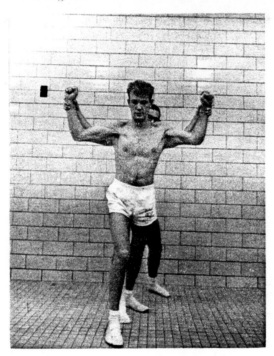

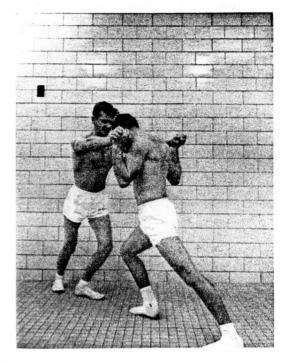

NOTE:

Exercises 6 and 7 may also be done lying on the back for better stabilization. See pictures for illustration. Raise the arms sideward to 90 degrees and bend the elbows to 90 degrees with the palms up. Attempt to rotate the shoulders externally as your partner resists for six seconds.

8. Shoulder Scapular Abduction

a. Raise the arms forward to 90 degrees with the palms up facing your partner. Push your arms forward reaching as far as possible while keeping your stomach muscles tight. Step forward with one foot for stabilization.

b. Your partner grasps your hands and attempts to push your arms backward and your shoulder blades together, resisting for six seconds.

c. Your partner does the same exercise raising his arms forward to 90 degrees and his palms up facing his partner.

d. Resist for six seconds by grasping his hands and attempting to push his arms backward and his shoulder blades together.

e. Each man repeats the exercise three times.

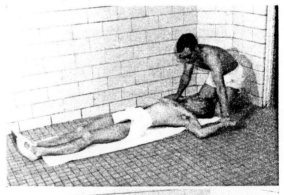

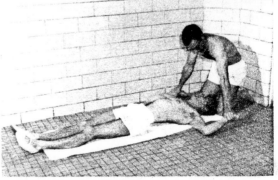

Attempt to rotate the shoulders internally as your partner resists for six seconds. Each man repeats the exercise three times. Exercise at three different positions through a complete range of motion in internal and external rotation.

9. Shoulder Scapular Abduction

a. Lying on your back, push your arms toward the ceiling stretching as far as possibile and keeping your elbows straight.

b. Your partner, with his body held rigid, balances his hips on your hands. Attempt to hold all of his body weight, resisting for six seconds.

c. Your partner does the same exercise pushing his arms toward the ceiling and attempting to hold all of your body weight.

d. Resist for six seconds.

e. Each man repeats the exercise three times.

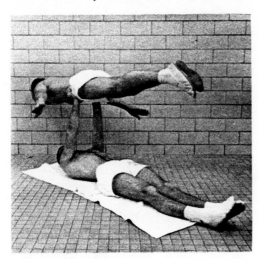

10. Elbow Flexion

a. Bend your elbows to 90 degrees bringing the palms toward your shoulders. Keep your stomach muscles tight. Bend the knees slightly for balance.

b. Your partner grasps your hands and attempts to straighten your elbows, resisting for six seconds.

c. Your partner does the same exercise bending his elbows to 90 degrees with the palms up.

d. Resist for six seconds attempting to straighten his elbows.

e. Each man repeats the exercise three times.

f. Exercise at three different positions through

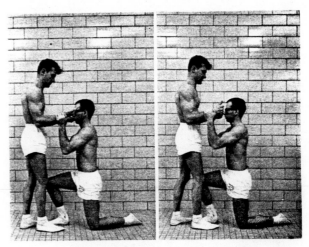

a complete range of motion in elbow flexion—45 degrees, 90 degrees, as shown in the picture, and at 135 degrees.

NOTE:

Exercise 10 should also be done by bringing the thumb toward the shoulder and by bringing the back of the hand toward the shoulder. Resistance is given the same way. Each man repeats the exercise three times each way. Exercise at three different positions through a complete range of motion in elbow flexion.

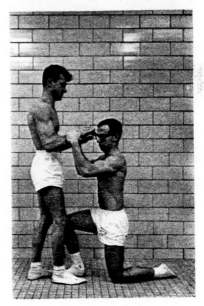

11. Elbow Extension

a. With your back to your partner, raise your arms directly overhead with the elbows bent slightly behind your head.

b. Bend your knees slightly for balance. Keep your stomach muscles tight.

c. Your partner grasps your wrists and attempts to prevent you from straightening your elbows, resisting for six seconds.

d. Your partner does the same exercise raising his arms directly overhead with the elbows slightly bent.

e. Resist for six seconds to prevent him from straightening his elbows.

f. Each man repeats the exercise three times.

g. Exercise at three different positions through a complete range of motion in elbow extension—135 degrees, 90 degrees, as shown in the picture, and at 15 degrees.

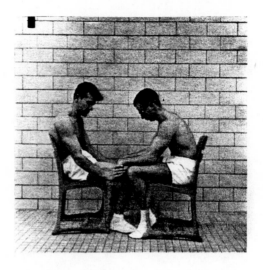

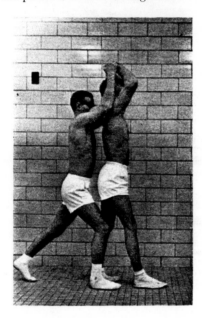

Wrist Exercises

1. Wrist Extension

a. Sit facing your partner with your forearms resting on your thighs for stabilization, the back of your hands up toward the ceiling, wrists held down just beyond your knees.

b. Partner sitting facing you attempts to push your hands down while you resist for six seconds.

c. Partner sits with the backs of his hands toward the ceiling.

d. You attempt to push his hands down while he resists for six seconds.

e. Each man repeats the exercise three times.

2. Wrist Flexion

a. Sit facing your partner with your forearms resting on your thighs, with the palm of your hands up toward the ceiling, wrists held down just beyond your knees.

b. Partner sitting facing you attempts to push your hands down while you resist for six seconds.

c. Partner sits with the backs of his hands toward the ceiling.

d. You attempt to push his hands down while he resists for six seconds.

e. Each man repeats the exercise three times.

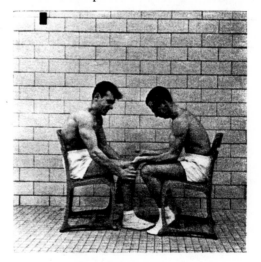

3. Wrist Abduction

a. Sit facing your partner with your forearms resting on your thighs, with the thumbs toward the ceiling, wrists held straight just beyond your knees.

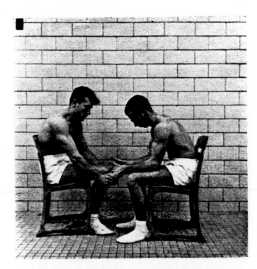

b. Partner sitting facing you attempts to push your hands down while you resist for six seconds.

c. Partner sits with the thumbs toward the ceiling.

d. You attempt to push his hands down while he resists for six seconds.

e. Each man repeats the exercise three times.

4. Wrist Adduction

a. Sit facing your partner with your forearms resting on your thighs, with the thumbs toward the ceiling, wrists held straight just beyond your knees.

b. Partner sits facing you and attempts to push your hands up toward the ceiling while you resist for six seconds.

c. Partner sits with the thumbs toward the ceiling.

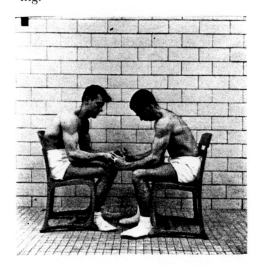

d. You attempt to push his hands upward while he resists for six seconds.

e. Each man repeats the exercise three times.

NOTE:

The four wrist exercises can be given without a partner by providing your own resistance with each hand. Repeat each exercise three times with six-second contractions and six seconds of rest between each exercise.

5. Wrist Pronation (Turning Palms Down)

a. Sit facing your partner. Extend your arms with the palms up.

b. Partner sitting facing you crosses his hands and grips your hands resisting you for six

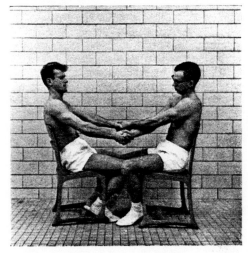

seconds. You try to turn your hands over to see the back of your hands.

c. Partner sits with his palms toward the ceiling.

d. Cross your hands and grip his hands. Resist his turning his hands over for six seconds.

e. Each man repeats the exercise three times.

6. Wrist Supination (Turning Palms Up)

a. Sit facing your partner. Extend your arms with the palms down.

b. Partner sitting facing you crosses his hands and grips your hands. You attempt to turn your hands over to bring your palms up; partner resists for six seconds.

c. Partner sits with the back of his hands toward the ceiling.

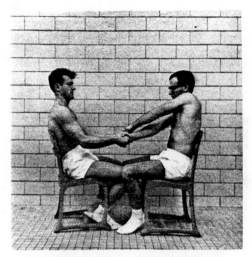

d. Cross your hands and grip his hands. Resist his turning the palms up for six seconds.

e. Each man repeats the exercise three times.

Finger and Hand Exercises

1. A Word of Caution

a. Do not use the Ed Block Hand Exercises following a serious hand injury or fracture unless prescribed by your physician.

b. This is a strenuous exercise program; stop exercising when your muscles become fatigued.

c. Like all exercise programs, begin with just a few exercises on the first few days.

d. You will get some muscle soreness in the fingers, wrists and forearms.

2. Procedure for the Whole Hand

a. Hold the putty in one hand.

b. Squeeze the putty with the whole hand; hold it tightly for six seconds; relax.

c. Squeeze the putty in the other hand; hold it tightly for six seconds; relax.

d. Squeeze the putty three times in each hand.

3. Procedure for the Individual Fingers (Finger Flexors)

a. Hold the putty in one hand.

b. Squeeze the putty between the tips of the index finger and the thumb; squeeze tightly for six seconds; relax.

c. Squeeze the putty between the tips of the middle finger and the thumb; squeeze tightly for six seconds; relax.

d. Repeat the exercise using each finger and thumb, holding for six seconds.

e. Exercise the other hand following the same procedure.

4. Procedure for the Individual Fingers (Finger Extensors)

a. Hold the putty in the palm of the hand.

b. Dig the fingernails and tips of the fingers into the putty.

c. Slowly try to straighten the fingers, one finger at a time, pushing against the putty.

d. Repeat the exercise three times with each finger.

e. Exercise the other hand following the same procedure.

5. Continuing Procedure

a. Carry your exerciser with you.

b. Exercise only once a day for the first few days.

c. After the initial muscle soreness subsides, you may exercise as often as you like to increase your hand, finger and wrist strength.

d. Strong hands are a must in all sports.

Finger and Hand Exercises

Strong hands are an asset in all sports. Playing the game of baseball will not give you strong hands. To gain strength and maintain muscle strength, we must load the muscles. That is, we must make the muscles work harder than they do in normal activity to gain strength. For this reason we must exercise our fingers, hands and wrists.

There are many hand exercisers on the market, but one of the best exercisers is an "Ed Block Hand Exerciser." This exerciser may be purchased from Skill Surgical, Inc., 3117 Green Mount Avenue, Baltimore, Maryland, 21218. The price is $1.80. See picture above.

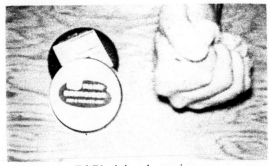

Ed Block hand exerciser.

All baseball players should have one of these exercisers and exercise with it every day. Follow the hand and finger exercises listed on the preceding page.

Chest Exercises

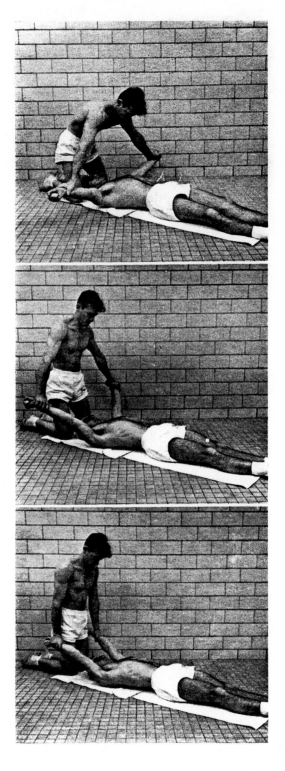

1. **Pull Your Arms Straight Across Your Chest (Back Lying)**
   a. Raise your arms out to the side to 90 degrees with your elbows straight and your palms up.
   b. Your partner grasps your wrists and attempts to hold the backs of your hands to the ground or floor as you lift your arms to go across your chest, resisting for six seconds. Keep your elbows straight.
   c. Your partner does the same exercise lifting his arms to go across his chest as you attempt to hold the backs of his hands to the ground or floor, resisting for six seconds.
   d. Each man repeats the exercise three times.
   e. Exercise at three different positions through a complete range of motion—at 15 degrees, 45 degrees, as shown in the picture, and at 90 degrees, with the arms perpendicular to the chest.

2. **Pull Your Arms Towards Your Opposite Hip (Back Lying)**
   a. Raise your arms overhead to a 45 degree angle with your elbows straight, palms up and the backs of the hands on the ground or floor.
   b. Your partner grasps your wrists and attempts to hold the backs of your hands on the ground or floor as you pull across your chest toward your opposite hip, resisting for six seconds.
   c. Your partner does the same exercise lifting his arms to go across his chest toward his opposite hip, resisting for six seconds.
   d. Each man repeats the exercise three times.
   e. Exercise at three different positions through a complete range of motion—at 15 degrees, 45 degrees, as shown in the picture, and at 90 degrees, with the arms perpendicular to the chest.

3. **Pull Your Arms Straight Down Towards Your Hips (Back Lying)**
   a. Raise your arms directly overhead with your elbows straight, palms up and the backs of the hands on the ground or floor.
   b. Your partner grasps your wrists and attempts to hold the backs of your hands to the ground as you lift your arms to go down to your sides, resisting for six seconds. Keep your elbows straight.
   c. Your partner does the same exercise lifting his arms to bring them up and to his sides, resisting for six seconds.
   d. Each man repeats the exercise three times.
   e. Exercise at three different positions through a complete range of motion—at 15 degrees, 45 degrees, as shown in the picture, and at 90 degrees, with the arms perpendicular to the chest.

Abdominal Exercises

1. V Sit-up (Back Lying)

   a. Raise both legs and your upper body simultaneously, keeping your legs straight with arms out straight for balance.

   b. Your partner attempts to push your back and legs to the ground, resisting for six seconds.

   c. Your partner does the same exercise lifting the upper body and the legs. Your arms are raised in front of your body for balance.

   d. Resist for six seconds.

   e. Each man repeats the exercise three times.

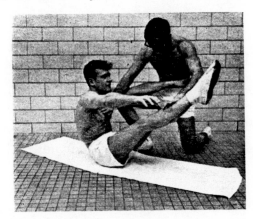

2. Bent Knees Sit-up (Back Lying)

   a. Raise the upper body off the ground in a half sit-up position with the hips and knees bent, feet on the ground near your buttocks, fingers laced behind your head.

   b. Your partner sits on your feet and holds your knees for stabilization while pushing on your chest or elbows, resisting for six seconds.

   c. At the end of the six-second contraction, continue the sit-up, touching the chest to the

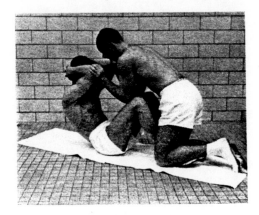

knees. Slowly return to the back lying position.

   d. Your partner does the same exercise while you attempt to push him back towards the ground, resisting for six seconds. Continue the sit-up, touching the chest to the knees. Slowly return to the starting position.

   e. Each man repeats the exercise three times.

3. Straight Leg Sit-up

   a. Raise the upper body off the ground in a half sit-up position with the legs out straight, fingers laced behind your head.

   b. Your partner sits on your legs for stabilization while pushing on your chest or elbows, attempting to push your back towards the ground, resisting for six seconds.

   c. At the end of the six-second contraction, con-

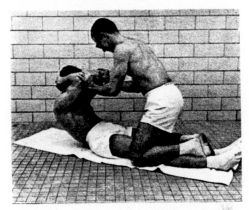

tinue the sit-up, touching the elbows to the knees. Slowly return to the back-lying position.

   d. Your partner does the same exercise while you attempt to push his back toward the ground, resisting for six seconds. Continue the sit-up, touching the chest to the knees. Slowly return to the starting position.

   e. Each man repeats the exercise three times.

4. Lateral Sit-up (Side Lying)

   a. Lie on your right side with your right arm across your chest. The left arm is raised to the side for balance.

   b. Your partner sits straddling your thighs for stabilization.

   c. Raise the upper body off the floor laterally as high as possible.

   d. Your partner attempts to push you down

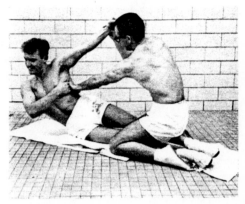

toward the ground with his hand on the side of your chest, resisting for six seconds.

e. Your partner does the same exercise while you attempt to push his upper body to the ground, resisting for six seconds.

f. Each man repeats the exercise on each side three times.

Back Exercises

1. Shoulder Hyperextension

a. Face lying, raise your arms as high as possible with the elbows straight and your palms up.

b. Your partner sits straddling your thighs.

c. Your partner attempts to push your arms to the ground, resisting for six seconds.

d. Your partner does the same exercise while you attempt to push his arms down, resisting for six seconds.

e. Each man repeats the exercises three times.

f. Exercise at three different positions through a complete range of motion in shoulder hyperextension—at 15 degrees, as shown in the picture, 45 degrees and at complete shoulder hyperextension.

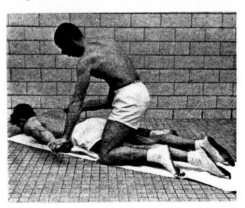

2. Shoulder Hyperextension (Shoulder Blade Pinched)

a. Face lying, pinch your shoulder blades together tightly and raise your arms as high as possible with the elbows straight and your palms up.

b. Your partner sits straddling your thighs.

c. Your partner attempts to push your arms to the ground, resisting for six seconds. Keep your shoulder blades pinched tightly.

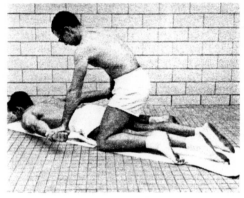

d. Your partner does the same exercise while you attempt to push his arms down, resisting for six seconds.

e. Each man repeats the exercise three times.

f. Exercise at three different positions through a complete range of motion in shoulder hyperextension—at 15 degrees, as shown in the picture, 45 degrees and at complete range of motion in shoulder hyperextension.

3. Scapular Adduction (Lift Arms Toward the Ceiling)

a. Face lying, raise the arms out to the side to 90 degrees. Rotate the arms externally with the thumb pointing upward toward the ceiling.

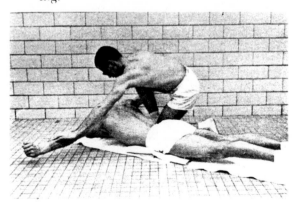

b. Your partner sits straddling your low back or kneeling beside your body.

c. Raise your arms as high as possible, leading with your thumbs while pinching your shoulder blades together.

d. Your partner attempts to push your arms down with his palm on your wrists, resisting for six seconds.

e. Your partner does the same exercise while you attempt to push his arms down, resisting for six seconds.

f. Each man repeats the exercise three times.

g. Exercise at three different positions through a complete range of motion in scapular adduction.

4. Shoulder Flexion

a. Face lying, raise the arms overhead to an angle of 45 degrees with your elbows straight and the back of your hands towards the ceiling.

b. Your partner is kneeling in front, near your head.

c. Raise your arms with the elbows straight and off the ground as high as possible while keeping your forehead on the ground.

d. Your partner attempts to push your arms down with his palms on the back of your hands and wrists, resisting for six seconds.

e. Your partner does the same exercise while you attempt to push his arms down, resisting for six seconds.

f. Each man repeats the exercise three times.

g. Exercise at three different positions through a complete range of motion in shoulder flexion.

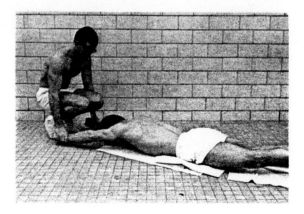

5. Back Hyperextension

a. Face lying, raise the head and chest off the ground as high as possible with the fingers laced behind your head.

b. Your partner sits straddling your thighs for stabilization.

c. Your partner attempts to push your chest toward the ground, resisting for six seconds.

d. Your partner does the same exercise while

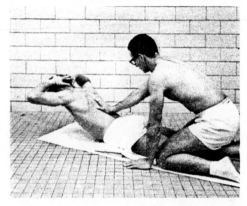

you attempt to push his chest toward the ground, resisting for six seconds.

e. Each man repeats the exercise three times.

f. Exercise at three different positions through a complete range of motion in back hyperextension.

6. Thigh Extension (Straight Leg Raising)

a. Face lying with the arms at the side of the body with the palms up.

b. Raise the leg off the ground just clearing the kneecap off the ground. Keep the knee straight and both hips on the ground.

c. Your partner is kneeling by your legs.

d. Your partner attempts to push your straight

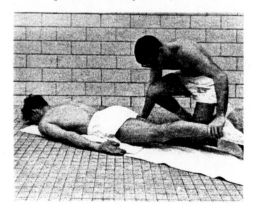

leg toward the ground, resisting for six seconds.

e. Your partner does the same exercise while you attempt to push his leg toward the ground, resisting for six seconds.

f. Each man repeats the exercise three times with each leg.

7. Thigh Extension (Straight Leg Raising)

a. Face lying with the arms at the side of the body with the palms up.

b. Raise the leg off the ground as high as possible, keeping the knee straight and both hips on the ground.

c. Your partner is kneeling by your legs.

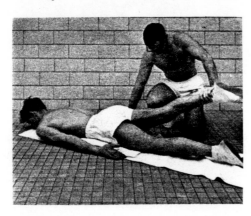

d. Your partner attempts to push your straight leg toward the ground, resisting for six seconds.

e. Your partner does the same exercise while you attempt to push his leg toward the ground, resisting for six seconds.

f. Each man repeats the exercise three times with each leg.

8. Thigh Extension (Bent Knee Leg Raising)

a. Face lying with the arms at the side of the body with the palms up.

b. Bend one knee and lift the bent knee off the ground as high as possible, keeping both hips on the ground.

c. Your partner is kneeling by your legs.

d. Your partner attempts to push your thigh toward the ground, resisting for six seconds.

e. Your partner does the same exercise while you attempt to push his thigh toward the ground, resisting for six seconds.

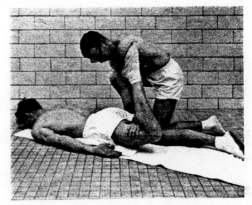

f. Each man repeats the exercise three times with each leg.

Hip Exercises

1. Hip Abduction (Sideward Leg Raising)

a. Side lying, the lower leg is bent for stabilization. The top leg is held with the knee straight. Raise the straight leg as high as possible, rotating the leg inward so that you lead with your heel.

b. Your partner is kneeling by your hips.

c. Your partner attempts to push your leg down

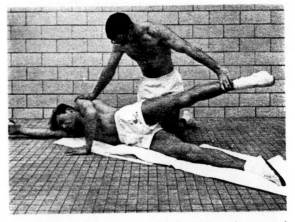

giving resistance at the knee for six seconds.

d. Your partner does the same exercise as you resist at the knee for six seconds.

e. Each man repeats the exercise three times with each leg.

f. Exercise at three different positions through a complete range of motion in hip abduction.

2. Hip Abduction (Sideward Leg Raising)

a. Side lying, the lower leg is bent for stabilization. The top leg is held with the knee

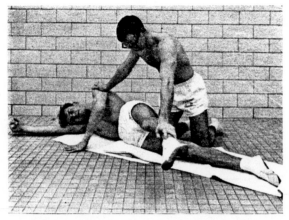

resist at the ankle for six seconds.

f. Each man repeats the exercise three times with each leg.

straight. The top leg is bent (flexed) at the hip to an angle of 45 degrees, keeping the knee straight.

b. Raise the top leg as high as possible, rotating the leg inward so that you lead with the heel.

c. Your partner is kneeling by your hip.

d. Your partner attempts to push your leg down giving resistance at the knee for six seconds.

e. Your partner does the same exercise as you resist at the knee for six seconds.

f. Each man repeats the exercise three times with each leg.

g. Exercise at three different positions through a complete range of motion in hip abduction.

3. Hip Flexion (Straight Leg Raising)

a. Back lying, raise the leg about 3 in. off the ground at the heel with the knee held straight. Your arms are held at the side.

b. Your partner is kneeling by your hips.

c. Your partner attempts to push your leg down, giving resistance at the ankle for six seconds.

d. Repeat the exercise with the other leg.

e. Your partner does the same exercise as you

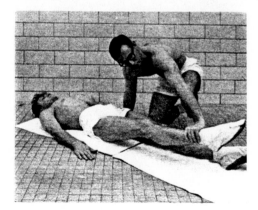

4. Hip Flexion (Straight Leg Raising)

a. Back lying, raise the leg to 45 degrees with the knee held straight. Your arms are held at the side. Your partner is kneeling by your hips.

b. Your partner attempts to push your leg down

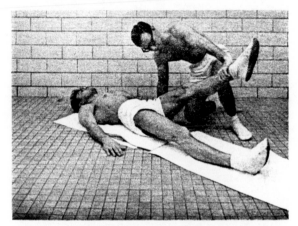

giving resistance at the ankle for six seconds.

c. Repeat the exercise with the other leg.

d. Your partner does the same exercise as you resist at the ankle for six seconds.

e. Each man repeats the exercise three times with each leg.

5. Hip Flexion (Knee Bent)

a. Sit on a table with the knees bent (flexed) to 90 degrees. A towel is rolled under the knees for comfort. The hands are on the outside of the knees, holding the table for stabilization.

b. Your partner is standing in front of your legs.

c. Raise your knee toward the ceiling keeping your knee bent.

d. Your partner attempts to push your leg down, giving resistance at the top of the knee for six seconds.

e. Repeat the exercise with the other leg.

f. Your partner does the same exercise as you resist at the knee for six seconds.

g. Each man repeats the exercise three times with each leg.

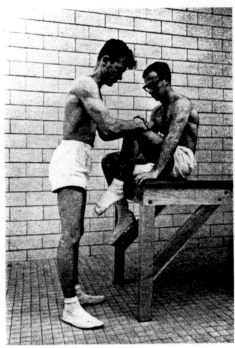

h. Exercise at three different positions through a complete range of motion in hip flexion.

6. Hip Flexion, Hip External Rotation and Knee Flexion

a. Sit on a table with the knees bent (flexed) to 90 degrees. A towel is rolled under the knees for comfort. The hands are on the out-

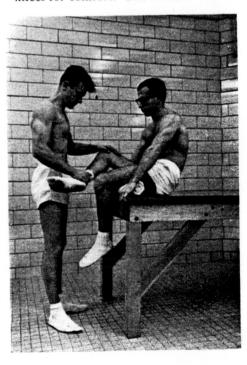

side of the knees, holding the table for stabilization.

b. Your partner is standing in front of your legs.

c. Raise your leg, attempting to cross your leg, rotating the hip externally and bringing the heel up along the shin of your opposite leg.

d. Your partner attempts to push your leg down, giving resistance with one hand on the top of your knee and the other hand grasping the ankle attempting to straighten your knee, resisting for six seconds.

e. Repeat the exercise with the other leg.

f. Your partner does the same exercise as you resist at the knee and ankle for six seconds.

g. Each man repeats the exercise three times with each leg.

h. Exercise at three different positions through a complete range of motion.

7. Hip Adduction (Hips and Knees Bent)

a. Back lying, your hips and knees are bent, (flexed) with the feet flat on the floor near your buttocks. Your arms are at the side of the body.

b. Your partner is kneeling by your hips.

c. Pull your knees together.

d. Your partner attempts to push your legs apart, giving resistance with one elbow wrapped around one knee and the other

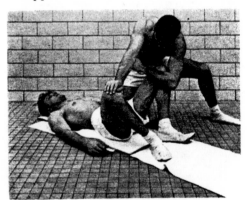

hand with the elbow straight against your other knee, resisting for six seconds.

e. Repeat the exercise three times, resisting for six seconds between each exercise.

f. Your partner does the same exercise as you resist at the knees for six seconds.

g. Each man repeats the exercise three times.

h. Exercise at three different positions through a complete range of motion.

8. Hip Adduction (Hips and Knees Straight)

a. Back lying, your legs are out straight and spread apart to about 45 degrees with your arms at the side.

b. Your partner is kneeling between your knees

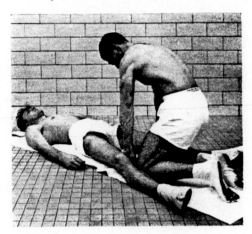

with his knees against the inside of your knees. *Do not resist at the ankles.*

c. Pull your legs together.

d. Your partner stops you from bringing your legs together, giving resistance with his knees for six seconds.

e. Repeat the exercise three times, resisting for six seconds between each exercise.

f. Your partner does the same exercise as you resist between the knees for six seconds.

g. Each man repeats the exercise three times.

NOTE:

Exercise number 8 should also be given with the legs spread about 3 in. and also spread about 6 in. to 8 in. apart at the knees. Resistance can be given with your two fists between your partner's knees. *Do not give resistance at the ankle as this will stretch the ligaments in the knee.*

Knee Exercises

1. Knee Extension

a. Sit on a table with the knees bent (flexed) over the edge of the table to 90 degrees. A towel is rolled under the knees for comfort. The hands are on the outside of the knees holding the table for stabilization.

b. Your partner is squatting in front of your legs. One hand is placed on the ankle, and the other hand is holding the leg of the table for stabilization.

c. Your partner holds your leg at 90 degrees while you attempt to extend your knee, resisting for six seconds.

d. Do not raise the buttocks or thigh off of the table during the exercise.

e. Repeat the exercises three times, resting for six seconds between each exercise.

f. Repeat the exercise three times with the other leg, or alternate exercising one leg and then the other leg.

g. Your partner does the same exercise as you resist at the ankle for six seconds.

h. Each man repeats the exercise three times with each leg.

2. Knee Extension

a. Sit on a table with the knee bent (flexed) over the edge of the table to 90 degrees. A towel is rolled under the knees for comfort. The hands are on the outside of the knees holding the table for stabilization.

b. Your partner is standing in front of your legs.

c. Raise one leg to 135 degrees.

d. Your partner attempts to push your leg down giving resistance at the ankle, for six seconds.

e. Do not raise the buttocks or thighs off of the table during the exercise.

f. Repeat the exercise three times, resting for six seconds between each exercise.

g. Repeat the exercise three times with the other leg, or alternate exercising one leg and then the other leg.

h. Your partner does the same exercise as you resist at the ankle for six seconds.

i. Each man repeats the exercise three times with each leg.

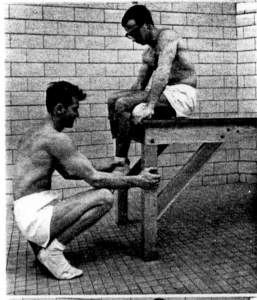

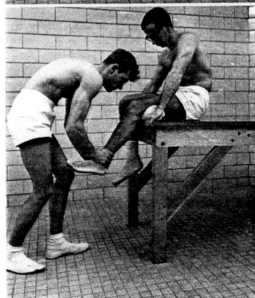

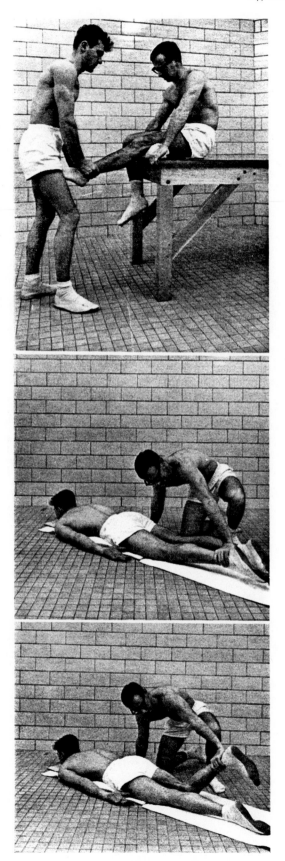

3. Knee Extension

a. Sit on a table with the knees bent (flexed) over the edge of the table to 90 degrees. A towel is rolled under the knees for comfort. The hands are on the outside of the knees holding the table for stabilization.

b. Your partner is standing in front of your legs.

c. Straighten your knee to about 165 degrees, 15 degrees off complete knee extension.

d. Your partner attempts to push your leg down giving resistance at the ankle for six seconds.

e. Do not raise the buttocks or thigh off the table during the exercise.

f. Repeat the exercise three times, resting for six seconds between each exercise.

g. Repeat the exercise three times with the other leg, or alternate exercising one leg and then the other leg.

h. Your partner does the same exercise as you resist at the ankle for six seconds.

i. Each man repeats the exercise three times with each leg.

4. Knee Flexion

a. Face lying, the arms are along the side of the body with the palms up, the legs out straight. Your partner is kneeling by your legs.

b. Bend one knee until your shin is about 3 in. off the ground or the floor. Keep both hips and both shoulders on the floor or the ground.

c. Your partner attemps to push your leg down, giving resistance at the ankle for six seconds.

d. Keep both hips and both shoulders on the floor during the exercise.

e. Repeat the exercise three times, resting six seconds between each exercise.

f. Repeat the exercise three times with the other leg, or alternate exercising one leg and then the other leg.

g. Your partner does the same exercise as you resist at the ankle for six seconds.

h. Each man repeats the exercise three times with each leg.

5. Knee Flexion

a. Face lying, the arms are along the side of the body with the palms up, the legs are out straight. Your partner is kneeling by your legs.

b. Bend one knee 135 degrees.

c. Your partner attempts to push your leg down, giv-

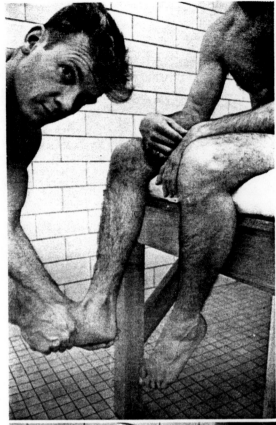

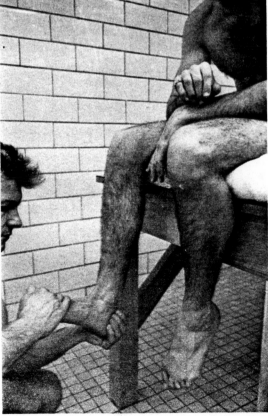

ing resistance at the ankle for six seconds.

d. Keep both hips and both shoulders on the floor during the exercise.

e. Repeat the exercise three times, resting six seconds between each exercise. Repeat the exercise three times with the other leg, or alternate exercising one leg and then the other leg.

f. Your partner does the same exercise as you resist at the ankle for six seconds.

g. Each man repeats the exercise three times with each leg.

Ankle Exercise

1. Ankle Inversion (Foot Turned In and Up)

a. Sit on a table with the knees bent (flexed) over the edge of the table to 90 degrees. A towel is rolled under the knees for comfort. The hands resting across the thighs.

b. Your partner is standing in front of your legs.

c. Raise your right leg to about 135 degrees. Push the foot down as far as possible.

d. Your partner places his left hand on the back of your right heel for stabilization. The right hand is placed on the inside of the right foot by the big toe.

e. Attempt to pull your right foot in and up, turning the sole of the foot to the inside. Your partner resists the attempt to pull your foot in and up for six seconds.

f. Repeat the exercise three times, resting six seconds between each exercise.

g. Repeat the exercise three times with the left ankle.

h. Reverse your hands for the left ankle with resistance given with the left hand.

i. Your partner does the same exercise as you resist at the ankle for six seconds.

j. Each man repeats the exercise three times with each ankle.

2. Ankle Dorsi-Flexion (Foot Pulled Straight Up)

a. Sit on a table with the knees bent (flexed) over the edge of the table to 90 degrees. A towel is rolled under the knees for comfort. The hands are resting across the thighs.

b. Your partner is standing in front of your legs.

c. Raise your right leg to about 135 degrees. Push the foot down as far as possible.

d. Your partner places his left hand on the back of your right heel for stabilization. The right hand is placed on the top of the foot and toes.

   e. Attempt to pull your right foot straight upward toward your face. Your partner resists the attempt to pull your right foot straight up for six seconds.

   f. Repeat the exercise three times, resting for six seconds between each exercise.

   g. Repeat the exercise three times with the left ankle.

   h. Reverse your hands for the left ankle with resistance given with the left hand.

   i. Your partner does the same exercise as you resist at the ankle for six seconds.

   j. Each man repeats the exercise three times with each ankle.

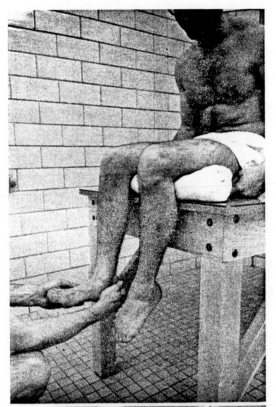

3. Ankle Eversion (Foot Turned Out and Up)

   a. Sit on a table with the knees bent (flexed) over the edge of the table to 90 degrees. A towel is rolled under the knees for comfort.

   b. Your partner is standing in front of your legs.

   c. Raise your right leg to about 135 degrees. Push the foot down as far as possible.

   d. Your partner places his right hand on the back of your right heel for stabilization. The left hand is placed on the outside of the right foot by the little toe.

   e. Attempt to pull your right foot out and up turning the sole of the foot to the outside. Your partner resists the attempt to pull your right foot out and up for six seconds.

   f. Repeat the exercise three times, resting six seconds between each exercise.

   g. Repeat the exercise three times with the left ankle.

   h. Reverse your hands for the left ankle with resistance given with the right hand.

   i. Your partner does the same exercise as you resist at the ankle for six seconds.

   j. Each man repeats the exercise three times with each ankle.

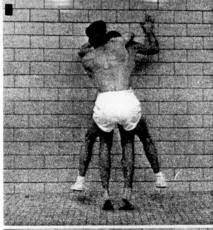

4. Ankle Plantar-flexion (Rise on the Toes)

   a. Stand with your back to your partner, with your feet 15 in. apart. Rise on your toes as high as possible keeping your back straight. Put your hands against the wall for stabilization.

   b. Your partner hangs his body weight on your shoulders, if possible, attempting to force your heels to the ground, resisting for six seconds.

   c. Your partner does the same exercise as you resist by hang-

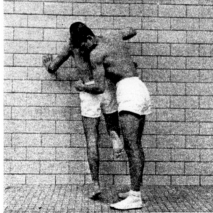

ing your body weight on his shoulders, resisting for six
seconds.

d. Each man repeats the exercise three times.

e. When beginning this exercise your partner may not be
able to take all of your weight. Begin with only part of
your weight and gradually add more weight.

NOTE:

Exercise 4 should also be done on one leg at a time. As your
strength increases, add more weight.

5. Ankle Plantar-flexion (Rise on the Toes with the Knees Bent)

a. Stand with your back to your partner, with your feet
about 15 in. apart. Do a half knee bend and rise on
your toes as high as possible, keeping your back
straight.

b. Keep your knees in a half knee bend position as you
rise on your toes.

c. Your partner hangs his body weight on your shoulders, if possible, attempting to force your heels to the
ground, resisting for six seconds.

d. Your partner does the same exercise as you resist by
hanging your body weight on his shoulders, resisting
for six seconds.

e. Each man repeats the exercise three times.

f. When beginning this exercise your partner will not
be able to take all of your weight. Begin with only
part of your weight and gradually add more weight.

NOTE:

Exercise 5 should also be done on one leg at a time. As
your strength increases, add more weight.

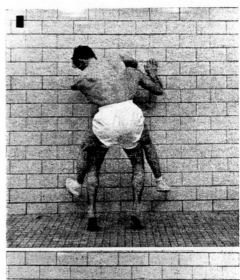

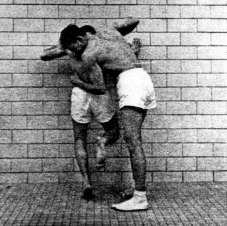

Pre-season Conditioning

THE USE OF SALT AND WATER

Drinking plenty of water and taking salt pills are very essential to all conditioning programs. All players who are working hard will sweat profusely. The heavier players may lose somewhere between 8 to 15 lbs. in a hard two-hour workout. They must drink plenty of water to replace this fluid loss and must also take salt pills to replace the salt. Most of this weight loss is fluid. Too many players have the false impression that in order to lose the excess weight that they picked up in the off-season, they must dehydrate the body and cut down on their fluid intake.

It is much better to lose a pound or two a day by burning up excess fatty tissue than to dehydrate the body. The body needs water and salt to keep its chemical balance. The physiology of salt and water balance in the body it too technical and complicated to explain in this book.

Salt helps the body retain some of the water, slows down the rate of fatigue and prevents muscle cramps and muscle strains or pulls. Water helps the body in the same way, plus preventing dehydration, heat exhaustion and heat stroke.

A working man needs water and salt. Coaches should stop practice several times in a two-hour or an hour-and-a-half workout to give the players water and salt pills. Fruit juices, cola drinks, water or any other fluids should be given, especially in hot weather with high humidity.

All athletes who are working out and sweating heavily should take a minimum of six to eight salt pills (five-grain) daily. The 225-lb. athlete who is losing 10 or more lbs. a workout should probably have more salt pills. Consult your team physician or team trainer for the amount of salt you should be taking. Do not take your salt pills all at one time before or after practice. Scatter your pills out throughout the day. Working out twice a day, it is a good idea to take two pills before practice, two after practice at both morning and afternoon workouts and two pills before going to bed.

It is good to supply the team with enteric-coated salt pills that do not break down quickly and cause some of the athletes to get nauseated. Some athletes find that salt pills make them sick. It is suggested that these athletes take their salt pills with their meals, and this will usually prevent such sickness.

If budgets permit, it is good to send each player a supply of enteric-coated salt pills with instructions on how he is to take them and how many pills he should take daily. The use of salt and plenty of water will prevent many pre-season and regular season injuries.

SPRINTING

Baseball players should never jog anywhere on the baseball field. If possible, your sprinting should be done outside with baseball shoes. Do as many sprints as you would under game conditions.

Too many baseball players try to get in shape by jogging a mile or two daily, thinking they are getting in good physical condition by increasing cardiovascular endurance. This is the wrong way to condition for baseball. All you are doing is getting in condition to jog a mile, two miles or even five miles. One sprint from home plate to third base on a triple, and this same man who can jog two miles cannot get his breath for five minutes.

Baseball is a game of many short sprints. Your body must be in condition to do many short sprints and respond quickly, so that you are ready for the next short sprint. Sprint like you do in the games. Take your stance at the plate, swing hard, and sprint 90 to 110 ft. as you would sprinting to first base. Repeat this sprint ten times.

Rest a few minutes; then swing hard, and sprint, rounding first base 180 to 200 ft. as you would hitting a double. Repeat this sprint ten times. Rest a few minutes or do some other exercises. Swing the bat hard and sprint, rounding first and second bases 270 to 300 ft. as you would hitting a triple. Rest a minute to a minute and a half and tag up as you would scoring on a fly ball, sprinting 90 to 100 ft. home.

How many times during the year do you see this winded player standing on third get thrown out at the plate trying to score on a fly ball? He has just hit a triple or run from first to third base on a single. In many cases this is just poor cardiovascular condition. Do not let this happen to you. Sprint every day to maintain good cardiovascular endurance.

Another sprint you should practice is taking a lead off first base and then sprinting 90 to 110 ft. to second base. Also, take a lead off first base and sprint, rounding second base as you do going from first to third base. This is the only way to sprint to condition for baseball. You should sprint three to five times daily during hitting practice during the regular season to maintain your speed and your footwork or skill rounding the bases.

Your turns or cutting rounding the bases put a lot of strain on your ankles and knees. Get your legs ready to do this for the season. Sprinting repeated 100-yd. dashes is fine, but this is not the type of sprinting you will be doing in the baseball games. Condition your body under game conditions and you will avoid or prevent many ankle and knee injuries.

Never jog anywhere or at any time while on the basefield. Sprint. Always try to sprint with someone faster than you are and keep up with him. When you sprint with someone slower than you are, you never sprint hard.

CATCHER

Catchers will condition as described previously for all baseball players. However, they will condition a little differently than the other positions when it comes to cardiovascular conditioning.

The catcher has to be in top condition due to the physical demands of catching. He is up and down hundreds of times during a game; he sprints to back up first base on every ground ball and to field bunts down the third and first base lines. Catching double headers is just twice as much work.

Have you ever noticed that most catchers are slow afoot and gradually lose more speed each year? Some of this loss of speed is considered an occupational hazard of catching. A catcher is squatting behind the plate most of the game and for hours at a time during spring training. With constant stretching of the quadriceps muscles in the front of the thigh, and the tightening or shortening of the hamstring muscles in the back of the thigh, he loses speed. With tight hamstring muscles, he cannot stretch out when he runs, and he has a shorter stride.

Running speed for the catcher can be maintained with a good stretching program. The catcher must stretch the muscles in the back of the legs (hamstrings) and the muscles of the low back. He must stretch these muscles daily in the off-season until he can lay his palms flat on the floor with the knees straight. It is necessary for him to continue this stretching daily throughout the season to be able to keep his palms flat on the floor. See hamstring stretch and shower-room procedure on pages 21 and 26.

The catcher should sprint daily as described earlier to maintain his speed year after year. Catchers should sprint with full equipment to get used to sprinting with equipment.

Practice the following sprints with your equipment on as you do in the games.

1. Take your position behind the plate. Throw off your mask, and sprint 90 to 100 ft. as you would to back up first base. Jog back and take your position behind the plate. Repeat this sprint until you are winded.

2. Take your catching position behind the plate. A partner will throw the ball in the air back by the screen about 60 ft. from home plate. Throw off your mask and sprint back to the screen as you would to catch a pop foul ball. This is one of the

hardest plays for the catcher. Repeat this sprint ten times.

3. Practice turning to your right and left going back for pop fouls. If you can find someone to fungo the ball high in the air, you can practice your sprinting and catching pop fly balls.

4. Practice fielding bunts down the third and first base lines. A partner will roll the ball down the third base line. Throw off your mask and sprint out to field the ball. Be in position to throw as you field the ball.

5. Your partner will role the ball down the first base line. Throw off your mask and sprint out to field the ball. It is not necessary to throw the ball when fielding bunts in pre-season conditioning. You will practice this same play many times and get plenty of throwing when practice or spring training begins.

6. The catcher will also play pepper games to help his fielding of short hops. Practice all your sprints and gradually increase the number of repetitions as your condition improves. The above sprints are just a few of the many sprints you can do to condition for baseball.

Sprinting repeat sprints to first, second and third base should also be done by the catcher. He must also build up endurance to sprint with full catching equipment since most of his sprinting will be done this way in the games.

The catcher will also continue his strength exercise with the weighted bat, medi exercise ball and isometric exercise in the pre-season program since he is the workhorse on the ball team. He should be sure to precede his sprinting with some warm-up exercises to stretch the body and get loose for sprinting. If the catcher follows this program, he should be ready for spring training in professional baseball, as well as university, high school or little league baseball.

PITCHER

Every player will condition a little differently to get ready to play his position. When early training begins, the pitchers will get a lot of help from the coaches or manager who always supervise the pitcher's conditioning program. In getting in condition in the off-season and pre-season, however, he must do a lot of strengthening, stretching and cardiovascular conditioning on his own as described for all baseball players.

In pre-season conditioning, the pitcher should get outdoors and run on the ground as soon as weather permits. He should dress warmly and wear baseball shoes to get used to running in them and to get his feet ready for the long season. Like all positions in baseball, the only way to get into condition is to sprint.

He must be able to sprint to cover first base, make the put out and come back to the mound and pitch. He must be in condition to come back and pitch without being winded and lose his control. The pitcher has to have great cardiovascular condition and strength to be able to pitch nine innings, back up every base for a possible overthrow and cover first base on balls hit to the first baseman. The physical demands on the pitcher are much greater than those on any other position.

All sprinting and throwing should be done as close to game conditions as possible. In preseason conditioning, here are a few sprints all pitchers should do. Begin slowly and do only a couple of each sprint drills the first few days. Increase the repetitions daily as your condition improves.

1. From your stretch position with a runner on first base, toss a ball easily and break for the first base line as you would fielding a bunt. A partner will roll the ball along the first base line to practice your fielding. Practice this drill until you are winded.

2. From both the stretch and a wind up, toss a ball easily and break for the third base line as you would to field a bunt. A partner will roll the ball down the third base line. Field the ball and practice your pivot to turn and throw to third base. Also practice your turn to throw to first base. It is not necessary to throw the ball in pre-season conditioning. You will get plenty of practice throwing when spring training or

school practice begins using the same drills.

3. Take your windup, toss the ball easily, and sprint to cover first base. A partner will throw the ball to you. Practice the play correctly hitting the base and turning into the infield ready to make another play. Repeat this drill ten times or until you are winded.

4. From a stretch position, toss the ball easily and sprint 90 ft. as you would to back up third base for a possible overthrow. Be in position to make a play and field the ball. Repeat this drill ten times.

These are just a few of the possible sprint drills. All coaches will have a few favorite drills. Practice sprinting to make all the possible plays you will make from the mound.

When spring training or practice begins in school, you will have many more drills like the ones described. You will also have the usual sprinting from foul line to foul line along the fence in the outfield. Usually you sprint one way and walk back on your heels with the ball of the foot off the ground. This exercise does a lot to prevent shin splints from running on your toes and to prevent overstretching the muscles along the front of the shin. By walking on your heels with the toes and ball of the foot off the ground, you can stretch the tight heel cords. See heel cord stretching exercises on page 27. Coaches and managers will also hit fungos for pitchers to sprint after.

Pepper games are great pre-season and regular season conditioning drills for all pitchers. To help pitchers with their fielding and reflexes, the hitter should be at least 60 ft. away in the pepper games and should hit the ball hard on the ground. This helps the pitcher to be ready always to field the hard-hit ball right back at him.

Pitchers will also play a lot of pick-ups as described on page 16. Practice all these drills and you will be ready and in great condition when spring practice begins.

FIRST BASEMAN

Follow the off-season program and pre-season sprinting program for all baseball players. The first baseman will have infield drills in fielding and throwing by the hour when practice begins. To make the drills easy, he should do many repeat short sprints in the same way that he will make the plays in the game.

Practice the following sprints with a partner to improve your cardiovascular condition.

1. A partner will roll the ball slowly in front of you so that you will have to sprint in hard as you do to field bunts and slow-hit balls. Field the ball in position to throw.

2. A partner will throw the ball on the ground to your right so that you will have to sprint or scoot after the ball. Stay low and field the ball in position to throw.

3. A partner will throw the ball on the ground to your left down the foul line so that you will have to sprint hard to field the ball.

4. Partner will throw the ball over your head to your right as a short pop fly into right field. Sprint hard into right field to make the catch.

5. Partner will throw the ball over your head to your left down the foul line as a short pop fly into right field. Sprint hard down the foul line to make the catch.

6. Partner will throw the ball directly over your head into right field. Sprint hard into right field to make the catch.

7. Partner will throw the ball in the air in foul territory as a pop fly in front of the dugout, half way between home plate and first base. Sprint in hard to make the catch.

8. Partner will throw the ball in the air as a pop fly over the pitcher's mound. Sprint in hard to make the catch.

Your partner will throw or roll the ball to a different spot each time. Field the ball, return to your regular position, and be ready to sprint in any direction to field the next ball. Begin with a few repetitions of each sprint, gradually increasing the number of sprints until you are in good physical condition. Spend some time every day stretching your shoulders, back and hamstrings (back of the legs).

It is not necessary to throw the ball after sprinting to field ground balls in your pre-season conditioning program. All you are interested in now is getting your cardiovascular condition and your legs in shape for the long season. As soon as practice or spring training begins, you will get all the throwing you need in many of the same drills. Playing pepper games is also a great conditioner for the first baseman.

SECOND BASEMAN

The cardiovascular demands for all infielders are very much the same in the short sprints to the bases, fielding ground balls and back into the outfield for short fly balls. The second baseman and the shortstop usually have more running than the other infielders in a ball game. They should be in excellent physical condition when practice begins. Spring training for the professional baseball player and practice for the school players was designed to perfect your skills and to teach you new ones.

After following the off-season program of strength and stretching exercises, here are a few sprints to improve your cardiovascular condition. Get your body ready for all the twisting, turning and short sprints you, as second baseman, will have to make.

Practice the following sprints with a partner who will throw or roll the ball far enough ahead of you to make you sprint hard to field the ball.

1. Partner will roll the ball slowly so that you will have to sprint in hard as you would to field slow-hit balls. Field the ball in position to throw to first base.

2. Partner will throw the ball on the ground to your right over second base so that you have to sprint after the ball. Stay low and field the ball in position to throw. Infielders always stay low and scoot after the ground balls.

3. Partner will throw the ball on the ground to your left between first and second base. Scoot after the ball as you field it.

4. Partner will throw the ball over your head into short center or right field as a short pop fly. Sprint back quickly to make the catch.

5. Partner will throw the ball over your head behind first base and down the foul line as a short pop fly. Sprint back quickly and make the catch.

6. Partner will throw the ball directly over your head into short right field. Sprint back quickly and make the catch.

7. Sprint to first base from your regular fielding position as you would to cover first base on bunts. Your partner will throw the ball to you when you get to the base.

8. Sprint to cover second base as you do on the double play. Your partner will throw the ball to you so that you can practice your pivots you will make on the double play.

Your partner will throw or roll the ball to a different spot each time. Field the ball, return to your regular position, and be ready to sprint in any direction to field the next ball.

It is not necessary to throw the ball after each sprint. Many boys will be working outside in cool or cold weather in the North before practice or spring training begins. It is much better to do your sprinting outdoors if possible with your baseball shoes. In the North in very cold weather, however, you may have to begin your sprinting indoors in the gym or fieldhouse.

Protect your arm; you will get plenty of throwing when practice or spring training begins in warm weather. Begin slowly with a few repetitions of each sprint drill. Increase the number gradually as your cardiovascular condition improves.

SHORTSTOP

The shortstop and second baseman will probably have more sprinting to do in the game than the other two infielders. The shortstop must back up bases for the possible overthrow; sprint to the outfield to act as relay man on balls hit between the outfielders or down the foul line; make the double plays at second base; and sprint for the ball between short and third base to make the tough play. The shortstop must be in excellent physical condition. Running speed, quick reflexes and a strong throwing arm are essential for a good shortstop.

Work with a partner who will throw or roll the ball far enough ahead of you to make you sprint and field the ball. Practice the following sprints to improve your cardiovascular condition.

1. Partner will roll the ball slowly toward you so that you will have to sprint in hard as you do to field slow-hit balls. Field the ball in position to throw.

2. Partner will throw the ball on the ground to your right in the hole between short and third base so that you will have to sprint hard to field the ball. Stay low, scoot after the ball, and field the ball in position to throw.

3. Partner will throw the ball on the ground over second base. Practice staying low and scooting after the ball as you field the ball.

4. Partner will throw the ball over your head into short center or left field as a short pop fly. Sprint back after the ball and make the catch.

5. Partner will throw the ball over your head behind third base and down the foul line as a short pop fly. Sprint back quickly to make the catch.

6. Partner will throw the ball directly over your head into short left field. Sprint back quickly to make the catch.

7. Partner will throw the ball in the air over the pitcher's mound as a pop fly so that you will have to sprint in hard to make the catch.

8. Sprint to second base from your regular position as you do to make the double play. Your partner will throw the ball to you to practice your pivot. Practice all the different pivots you will make on the double play.

It is not necessary to throw the ball on every sprint drill or double play, as you will get plenty of throwing when practice begins. Your partner will throw or roll the ball to a different spot each time. Field the ball, return to your regular position, and be ready to sprint in any direction to field the next ball.

Practice each sprint a few times. Begin slowly with a few repetitions, and gradually increase the number of repetitions as your condition improves. Play pepper games daily to help your fielding and reflexes.

UTILITY INFIELDERS

Utility infielders and utility outfielders will condition in the off-season as recommended for all players. They should condition in pre-season as recommended for the second baseman and shortstop, as these two positions require more cardiovascular conditioning than the other two infield or outfield positions.

Utility men in professional baseball have a difficult time staying in condition during the season. Gaining weight is always a big problem. They must watch their weight, diet, pitch batting practice, continually have the coach hit ground balls to them, exercise, stretch daily to maintain their flexibility and strength and sprint every day. They must stay in condition so that they are ready to play whenever the manager or coach needs them at any time during the season. Pepper games are also good for the utility infielder.

THIRD BASEMAN

The third baseman, like all infielders, must be in good physical condition to make the difficult plays required of him. Cardiovascular condition is the most difficult to acquire and to maintain over the long season. To acquire cardiovascular condition, he, too, must do many repeat short sprints.

Work with a partner who will throw or roll the ball far enough ahead of you to make you sprint and field the ball. Practice the following sprints to improve your condition.

Take your regular fielding position.

1. With the bunt in order, your partner will roll the ball slowly down the foul line as you sprint in to field the bunt.

2. Partner will roll the ball slowly to your left in front of the shortstop as you sprint to field the ball. Field the ball in position to throw.

3. Partner will throw the ball hard to your left in front of the shortstop as you sprint

hard to make the play. Field the ball in position to throw.

4. Partner will throw the ball hard on the ground to your right down the foul line as you scoot to your right to field the ball. Field the ball in position to throw.

5. Partner will throw the ball over your head down the left field foul line in foul territory as a short foul fly ball. Sprint down the foul line and make the catch.

6. Partner will throw the ball in the air in foul territory as a pop fly in front of the dugout, halfway between third base and home plate. Sprint in hard to make the catch.

Your partner will throw the ball to a different spot each time. Make the catch or field the ground ball and return to your fielding position. Be ready to sprint in any direction. Repeat the sprints until you are winded and cannot sprint for another ball. Rest a few minutes and sprint again. As your cardiovascular condition improves, you will be sprinting much longer before getting winded. Gradually increase the number of sprints until you are in good physical condition.

After a good off-season strength and stretching program and a good pre-season sprint program, you will be ready to play the first day of practice or spring training.

When spring training begins, you will do many more sprint drills and field ground balls by the hour. Play pepper games with the other infielders.

OUTFIELDER

Running speed and a strong throwing arm are the prerequisites for a good outfielder. The outfielder must make longer sprints than the infielders. He must also sprint to back up all bases for possible overthrows. On all plays in the field, the outfielder should be sprinting in to back up the play. The outfielder will sprint to back up the other outfielders on all fly balls and all ground balls.

If possible, work with a partner who will throw the ball far enough ahead of you to make you sprint hard to catch the ball. Practice the following sprints. Take your regular fielding position ready to sprint in any direction.

1. Sprint to your right at least 90 ft.: your partner will throw the ball in front of you with enough lead to make you sprint hard to make the catch.

2. Sprint to your left for 90 ft.; your partner will throw the ball in front of you to make you sprint as fast as you can to make the catch.

3. Partner will throw the ball over your head about 90 ft. as you sprint back to make the catch.

4. Partner will throw the ball 90 ft. in front of you as you would sprint in fast to catch a pop fly.

5. Sprint in fast as your partner throws the ball on a line as you would sprint in for a line drive. Make the catch and be in a position to throw.

6. Take your regular position. Your partner will throw the ball to a different spot each time. Make the catch and be ready to sprint in any direction.

7. Practice wearing baseball sun glasses to get used to flipping the glasses down when the flyball goes through the sun. Playing the sun field is very difficult for many outfielders.

When practice begins, a coach or manager will hit flyballs to you by the hour. It is better in pre-season for greater accuracy, to have someone throw the ball to you rather than fungo the ball, and you can do more sprinting. Begin with a few repetitions of each sprint. Gradually increase the number of sprints as your condition improves.

Outfielders should also play pepper games as the pitchers do to practice fielding ground balls. It is better to have the hitter stand at least 60 ft. away from the fielders and hit the ball hard. Ground balls that get by the outfielders are two- and three-base errors. Practice fielding ground balls. Outfielders should also play pick-ups as recommended for pitchers on page 16.

Seasonal Conditioning

BEFORE EVERY GAME

Baseball players should do something during the entire season to maintain their strength, speed, flexibility and cardiovascular endurance.

Before every game baseball players should do some warm-up and stretching exercises to get the body ready for the game. Always jog around the field to loosen up, gradually increasing your speed until you are loose enough to sprint. Use infield and outfield practice and batting practice to get loose for the game. Sprint hard several times after you are warmed up before every game.

In the clubhouse, use the weighted bat daily as described on page 28 to keep your wrist and forearms strong. Use your Ed Block Hand Exerciser to keep your hands strong. Stretch your shoulders, back and hamstrings (back of the legs) daily. Stay strong throughout the season to avoid injury. Take your salt pills daily.

DURING THE GAME

1. When the last out is made in an inning, sprint hard to the dugout. Always make it a point to beat the pitcher to the dugout. It is a good idea for managers and coaches to insist that all players do this.
2. When your side is out, sprint hard out to your position. By sprinting in and out from your position, you will always stay warm and will cut down your chances for muscle strains and pulls.
3. Use a fungo bat and stretch your shoulders and back well every time before you hit.

Never Walk on the Baseball Field — Sprint!

All baseball players should report to practice on the first day in good physical condition ready to play. Do not let an early injury due to poor physical condition keep you from making the team. Spring training or practice should be used to practice and improve your skills, to teach you new skills and to improve your timing.

TIPS ON CONDITIONING THE THROWING ARM

1. Be sure your legs are in good physical condition before you start throwing hard. Sprint daily.
2. Learn to use the body and legs in every throw. Coaches should teach every player how to throw correctly.
3. Do not throw hard until the stiffness and tired feeling from early season work is gone.
4. Never throw hard indoors. Usually you feel strong after not throwing all winter. Many arms are injured when the foot slips on a smooth gym floor.
5. Pitchers should throw only straight balls until the arm is strong and the weather is warm.
6. To practice your curve ball early, just spin the ball until the muscles get used to the curve ball motion. Do not try to break off a good curve until your arm is strong and your body is in good condition.
7. Wear wool shirts in the spring in cold or cool weather. Many professional baseball players wear a sweatshirt to bed early in the year so that the arm does not get chilled during the night and the muscles tighten up.
8. Do not stand around with a wet sweatshirt and supporter on after throwing or infield practice. Put on dry clothes and a rubber jacket. Finish every practice with sprinting.
9. Use analgesic balm on the low back, shoulders and elbows in cold weather. Always

wear long-sleeved sweatshirts until July or hot weather begins.

10. Buy a rubber jacket to protect your arm from the wind and cold weather.

11. At the first sign of a sore arm, tell your coach and trainer. You cannot throw a sore arm out as the old baseball saying goes. You need good treatment and rest for a sore arm. Find a good physician and a good trainer.

12. Turtle neck sweaters are used by many professional baseball players to keep the neck and shoulders warm in the spring. Most sporting goods stores sell turtle neck sweaters for baseball.

13. Never ride in a car with the window open or in a convertible without a jacket before or after pitching. All baseball players should wear a light jacket after playing. Keep your arm covered at all times.

14. Some pitchers and infielders have trouble with blisters on their finger tips early in the year. Use Tuf-skin or Benzoin to toughen the skin. Do not cut your finger nails too short.

15. After workouts, take a warm shower and cool off before going out in the cold. An Alcohol rub helps. Always wear a coat or jacket.

16. Today, air-conditioned hotels, buses, trains and planes are a problem. Always wear long-sleeved pajamas or a light sweatshirt to bed at night. Always wear a jacket when riding on air-conditioned buses, trains or planes. When you get chilled your muscles will get tight and may cause arm injuries.

Conclusion

Conditioning for baseball is a twelve-month job. Baseball players cannot allow themselves to get out of condition in the off-season. When baseball season ends in September or October, take a week or two off and rest. Then begin playing handball, swim, or participate in some other active sport to maintain your speed, agility, flexibility, strength and cardiovascular endurance.

Baseball players have a tendency to gain weight in the off-season due to a tremendous appetite during the season. Banquets in the off-season do not help the weight problem. Weigh yourself every morning when you get out of bed. Anytime you gain 5 lbs. above your playing weight, you should diet or push away from the table for a few days until you are back at your playing weight. It is much easier to lose weight this way than to wait until you are 20 lbs. overweight.

For the lightweight athlete in little league, high school, college and professional baseball, many physicians recommend Nutrament as a diet suplement to help gain weight. Each 12½-oz. can is a perfect balanced meal. Nutrament supplies a satisfying 400-calorie meal, with 20 gms. of protein, 13.3 gms. of fat and 50 gms. of carbohydrate, plus controlled amounts of all known essential vitamins and minerals. Nutrament is made by Edward Dalton Company, Evansville, Indiana, 47721.

To gain weight the athlete will drink two to three cans daily with his meals. It is recommended he drink one can with his lunch, one at dinner and one before he goes to bed. With his regular diet plus 1200 calories of Nutrament and good exercise, the athlete should be able to gain weight.

To be good at anything you have to work hard at it for twelve months out of the year. Keep in top physical condition and you will have a long baseball career.

Exercise Prescription

Name ....

Playing Weight ....

Strengthen Weak Areas — Do Exercises on Pages ....

....

....

Off-season — Do Exercises on Page ....

....

....

Pre-season — Continue Exercises on Page ....

....

....

Follow Cardiovascular Sprinting to Play ....

....

....

Index